Narratives of Recovery from Serious Mental Illness

William Tucker

Narratives of Recovery from Serious Mental Illness

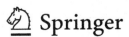 Springer

William Tucker
Columbia College of Physicians and Surgeons
New York, NY
USA

ISBN 978-3-319-33725-8   ISBN 978-3-319-33727-2   (eBook)
DOI 10.1007/978-3-319-33727-2

Library of Congress Control Number: 2016938657

Printed on acid-free paper

This Springer imprint is published by Springer Nature
The registered company is Springer International Publishing AG Switzerland

To Sheila, my anchor and my sail

Foreword

When a resident in psychiatry in the early 1970s, I was cautioned against working in a state mental hospital or clinic. The risk of doing so, I was told, was that I would become discouraged (and possibly leave the field) since none of my patients would get better. The prevailing view within my field and among the general public was that a serious mental illness, especially schizophrenia, ushers in a lifetime of disability and despair.

So while I took call at a state hospital I did not start working in public mental health until 2007 when I became chief medical officer of the largest state mental hospital system in this country. By then, not only had the bleak prospects for people with mental disorders come under great challenge I could dedicate myself to a growing ethos and clinical practice of recovery for those with persistent mental disorders, and their families.

Dr. Bill Tucker, who served in the same position I now do but for him some years ago, gives us a book meant to illustrate by case example, by individual stories, how lives with relationships, contribution, work, school, purpose and dignity can be restored to people with serious mental illnesses. He shows us and thereby fosters hope, by giving us the stories of twelve patients he personally treated, as part of a psychiatric outreach team in the community, in New York City. After working as a state official, Dr. Tucker literally rolled up his sleeves and took care of very ill patients under challenging and at times daunting circumstances. He hopes that his work will encourage others to put skepticism and stigma aside and discover the rewards of patient care outside the office and beyond the "worried well."

Recovery from serious mental illness is not a singular or monochromatic process. In an effort to define recovery, and thereby better refine an understanding of its approaches, colleagues and I described some of its dimensions, which are interlocking and certainly not mutually exclusive (Lieberman et al. 2008).

Recovery in patients with serious mental illness can and does occur in the biological substrates of the brain: growth of neural and glial (connective) cells is possible, cell loss (evidenced by brain grey matter reductions) can be attenuated;

neural connectivity and brain flow can be improved. Sensory gating can be improved. We are still learning more—especially about neurogenesis.

Recovery from acute psychosis is well known, especially for the so-called positive symptoms like hallucinations and delusions. Negative symptom recovery remains on the list of what our field needs to do more for.

Recovery of cognitive functions impacted by mental illness, especially schizophrenia, has advanced substantially in the past decade. These capabilities include attention, focus, memory and decision-making. Improvement in these areas is essential for people to function in their own self-care, autonomy, and capacities for school and work.

Recovery too of social functions is possible and our techniques to assist are continually improving. Social-skills training has become an integral part of psychiatric rehabilitation and re-opens the doors of human connection and relatedness that were too often lost with chronic mental illness.

With recovery, as well, the quality of a person's life improves, as does their ability to be a responsible agent, a decision-maker, in their own life. With these strengths comes the spirit of hope that recovery breeds and sustains.

Dr. Tucker does not oversell recovery. He does not understate the demands upon patient, family and clinician that the path of recovery requires: He is too good a doctor and he is an honest broker of the kind of effort needed to achieve success. But his work, his insights, his example, and his hope are welcome beacons of light in my field—which too often still lives in the shadows or does not get its message out as clearly as needed to overcome the doubters.

Recovery is possible for people with serious mental illness. You don't have to believe me. You just need to read this book.

New York City   Lloyd I. Sederer
December 2015   MD

Reference

Lieberman JA, Drake RE, Sederer LI et al (2008) Science and recovery in Schizophrenia. Psychiatr Serv 59(5)

Preface

I write this book to commemorate all my patients at Pathways to Housing from 2005 to 2011—not only those who recovered, because they all welcomed me into their lives and invited me to share in their efforts toward recovery. Its purpose is threefold: (1) to illustrate my view of the success of some of them with those efforts; (2) to suggest to policy-makers how outreach psychiatry can bridge the gap between institutional treatment or homelessness and stability in the community; and (3) to invite fellow psychiatrists at any stage of their careers to enter this work and improve on it.

Acknowledgements

I could not have begun without the guidance and encouragement over many years of Christian Beels and Marianne Eckardt. Kim Hopper and John Tepper-Marlin reviewed the manuscript and did their best to improve its accuracy and clarity. Janice Stern, my editor, is truly the midwife who brought it into the world.

Contents

Chapter 1
Introduction

What Is Recovery, and How Does It Relate to Stability?

Patient advocates describe recovery as achieving or returning to a life that encompasses the usual elements that people without serious mental illness also seek: decent housing, access to transportation, access to adequate general health care, opportunities for forming meaningful relationships, a sense of accomplishment, and, for some, gainful employment.

Psychiatrists, policy-makers, and community residents describe stability as maintaining oneself in an independent home environment, taking medications for both psychiatric and general systemic illnesses that are effective in preventing relapse or deterioration and tolerable in terms of side effects, attending a clinic or going to a primary-care physician for necessary health management and treatment, and avoiding repeated recourse to emergency services and hospitals.

These two descriptions are not identical, but they are entirely compatible and reinforce each other so nicely that it is hard to imagine one without the other. Recovery provides the motivation, and stability provides the means. This book illustrates both.

The problem is that people in transition from institutions or from the streets to living in the community are for the most part not ready to commit themselves to regular routines of management of their illnesses; therefore, the usual mental health clinic services are inadequate. What they need instead during this period are outreach services.

This book is aimed at addressing three obstacles to increasing such outreach services: public skepticism, limited funding, and scarcity of professionals interested in providing them. First, it offers a realistic account of the process of successful stabilization for 12 specific individuals living in the community and an illustration of what recovery involved for them; second, it addresses the obstacles that limit its wider implementation, so that policy-makers might consider supporting it through increased funding of such services, which provide the less expensive and more

© Springer International Publishing Switzerland 2016

W. Tucker, *Narratives of Recovery from Serious Mental Illness*,
DOI 10.1007/978-3-319-33727-2_1

humane alternative to continued institutionalization; and third, it may—just may— suggest, to mental health professionals at any stage of their careers, the possibility of engaging in this emotionally and intellectually rewarding work themselves, thereby acquiring the skills and experience they can use to refine the accounts that follow and to produce those of their own.

There are no new ideas here. The realization that recovery from serious mental illness was the general rule, rather than the rare exception, occurred to no less an authority on schizophrenia than Bleuler (1911); Assertive Community Treatment (ACT), the modality for promoting stability, was developed by Leonard Stein and Mary Ann Test over a third of a century ago (Stein and Test 1980); and the crucial update to this modality, namely, the provision of "housing first," which is particularly important in dense, urban environments, was combined with ACT services into a wrap-around treatment program over two decades ago by Tsemberis and Eisenberg (2000).

The message that recovery is the rule rather than the exception has been announced before (Davidson et al. 2005). A notable example that interweaves several accounts of recovery is presented in a history of Fountain House, a successful and well-known rehabilitation facility in New York City (Flannery and Glickman 1996). But in the mental health field generally, very few have heard this message, and still fewer have become convinced. Instead, the vast majority of mental health professionals do not accept that recovery is the rule, the recent case of the late John Nash notwithstanding. Their first reason is theoretical: toward the end of the nineteenth century, Emil Kraepelin, often referred to as "the founder of modern scientific psychiatry," conceptualized both common types of serious mental illness as leading to inevitable deterioration: the progressively deteriorating one, schizophrenia; and the relapsing one, manic-depressive illness, where the deterioration would be punctuated by transient periods of improvement (Kraepelin 1883). His concept has remained in force through the training of generations of mental health professionals, up to the present day. Three decades after Kraepelin's book, Bleuler famously described what he considered the core features of schizophrenia (the "four A's": ambivalence, autism, loosened associations, and blunted affect), which he felt never disappeared entirely. Toward the end of that same book he included his further observation that, "reports from clergymen and relatives…speak only occasionally of a true cure, although the majority of the released individuals are either employed or employable (Bleuler, p. 256)." However, this further observation, crucial to the argument for recovery, was never transmitted to later practitioners.

Their second reason is to some degree empirical: patients with these conditions are either lost to follow-up, as they wander back and forth between hospitals and community clinics, caught in the extremely expensive course euphemized by the press as the "revolving door" (Gladwell 2006); or they remain hospitalized indefinitely; or they recover so well and manage to blend into the general medical treatment system so successfully that they no longer interact with the public mental health system at all. In this scenario, mental health professionals do not realize they were ever seriously mentally ill in the first place and distrust the accounts their patients tell them about it—again, John Nash. Thus, the notion of recovery from serious mental illness usually meets with skepticism or with outright suspicion about the motives of someone who acknowledges it—for example, that she or he is exaggerating the virtues of some new pharmaceutical product that claims to produce it, as I was accused of doing.

In fact the countervailing view, that recovery is not only possible but is the usual outcome for the majority of people with serious mental illness, was demonstrated and reported half a century ago. Recovery is the theme of "The Vermont Story," a report to the American Public Health Association in 1962 of a project carried out by George Brooks and colleagues at the Vermont State Hospital. They describe how they first prepared, then discharged, and then followed up for 5 years, a cohort of several hundred patients who had been hospitalized there for an average of 10 years. Of those they discharged, only a small subset ever returned to the hospital. They noted that, while the medications developed in the prior decade made a significant contribution, the success of their program was also due to two other factors: first, to their optimism and their provision of suitable transitional housing ("they [i.e., the patients] would have had to be more out of contact with reality than they were, to want to exchange the security and comfort of the hospital for joblessness and no suitable place to live in the community [Eldred p. 45]"), and second, to the efforts of the patients themselves (they [i.e., the patients] were reluctant to fail those who had faith in them [Eldred p. 46]). A quarter of a century later, Harding contributed periodic, well-documented follow-up studies on this initial cohort and successive ones, in which she found that they had successfully blended into their respective communities and were living independently, earning incomes comparable to non-afflicted neighbors, and receiving treatment for residual symptoms from their primary-care providers, rather than from the public mental health system (Harding et al. 1987).

"That is all very well in rural Vermont," objected a group of sophisticated and thoughtful psychiatric residents from Bellevue to whom I was teaching community psychiatry in the mid-1990s during my tenure with the New York State Office of Mental Health (NYS-OMH), "but what would happen to such a group of patients released to the streets of New York, where housing is scarce, drugs are plentiful, and victimization is common?" That was a thoughtful challenge at the time, and many would raise it still.

What Is Serious Mental Illness?

"Serious Mental Illness" is a shortened version of "Serious and Persistent Mental Illness," which is what NYS-OMH defines as its core target population. It includes a number of diagnoses not envisioned by Kraepelin (Section "What Is Recovery, and How Does It Relate to Stability?") in his binary schema, but clearly defined in the Diagnostic and Statistical Manual, Third Edition, published in 1980, and in all subsequent editions, including the most recent one, DSM-V. These diagnoses include severe depression, the range of post-traumatic conditions, the group of severe personality disorders called "Cluster A," and, most importantly, all the chronic substance abuse disorders. Furthermore, it is intended to convey that diagnosis alone, based on symptoms, however severe, is insufficient for inclusion: there must be a disability component as well, usually involving multiple areas, such as interpersonal relationships, health, and work. All the subjects of the narratives here meet this definition, and they have experienced enormous suffering and stagnation besides.

Why We Need Expanded Outreach Services

Let me explain how mental health clinics usually function. Some decades ago, these clinics in New York State were required to have contracts with hospitals that guaranteed back-up emergency evaluation and, if necessary, rehospitalization, as a condition of their obtaining operating certificates. Such contracts provided hospitals with the leverage to require, in turn, that the referring clinics send a staff member along with the patient to provide first-hand information about the reason for the referral, the patient's level of functioning before the new symptoms arose, and the current treatment, including medications and social supports. These provisions, in turn, often made it possible to avoid extended stays in emergency rooms or in-patient units, since the clinic often wanted only a "second opinion" in order to deal with a change in symptoms or status that was the reason for referral. This reciprocity between clinic and emergency room enhanced the efficiency of the system enormously. When extended observation was required, appropriate modifications in treatment could begin immediately, since the patient's current treatment regimen was clear; thus, rehospitalization could be brief. Electronic medical records at best can provide only a partial substitute for the presence of a knowledgeable staff member, since they are only available if the referring clinic and the hospital share common software—by no means the usual situation; more importantly, they rarely describe the reason for the current referral.

But such contracts are no longer required for licensure, so the clinics can no longer be required by hospitals to send staff members along with the patients referred for evaluation. You might think that they would be motivated to do so, anyway, since it is obviously in the interest of the overall healthcare system to initiate appropriate treatment as soon as possible. But that is not how the system functions. Funding for each sector of the healthcare system is independent of that for the other sectors. Clinics are motivated to maximize billable treatment hours; thus, patients who do not show up for appointments represent a loss of income. Outreach takes time, even for a phone call, which is the most that typically occurs, and that time cannot be billed. On the other hand the open staff hours created by closed cases can easily be filled, either by scheduling new intakes or by asking already stable, treatment-adherent patients to increase the frequency of their visits; thus, no loss of income need result from closing the cases of problematic patients.

As a result, clinic administrators and their staffs are motivated to make emergency rooms the default option, should any threat to the patient's ongoing attendance occur, whether from lack of motivation, after-hours needs, or deterioration in status, as, for example, because of an acute medical problem. Hence the current lack of coordination between clinics and emergency rooms on the front end, and between hospitals and outpatient clinics on the back end.

However, as a result of recent Medicare policies that penalize hospitals for readmitting patients in certain diagnostic categories who return within a month of discharge, hospitals themselves have become motivated to try to ensure continuity with community care, as a means of reducing early readmissions. They have employed such interventions as engaging earlier with discharge planning in the course of a hospital stay, providing a month's supply of medication on discharge rather than only a prescription, and making at least one follow-up phone call after discharge to encourage the patient's attending the first scheduled follow-up visit. But these interventions are insufficient. Even within a single healthcare system, as I saw during my tenure at the NYS-OMH, inpatient and outpatient physicians did not discuss their respective medication prescribing policies, let alone agreeing upon them. For their part many patients, especially those recently released from institutional confinement, do not have comfortable, familiar relationships with community providers, nor do the providers themselves feel comfortable with them. For other reasons systems leaders themselves often fare no better. The Chief Medical Officer of a large, mid-western tertiary-care medical center explained to me that his hospital center, having performed a complex surgical procedure, such as a transplant, on a patient coming from a considerable distance, often cannot locate a generalist or specialty physician to refer the patient back to in her/his home community and therefore is likely to incur such penalties. Other physicians, patients, and concerned participants in our disjointed healthcare systems will be familiar with their own versions of this discontinuity.

Furthermore, many discharged patients may lack stable housing. Homelessness makes the management of any chronic illness almost impossible, starting with the simple requirement for a permanent address in order to refill a prescription. The principle of "housing first" was recognized early on in the provision of care for patients with HIV/AIDS, and it is equally indispensable for community stabilization for people with serious mental illness. Gladwell cites a careful study suggesting that only 10 % of the homeless population is chronically homeless, and thus in need of being provided with suitable and acceptable housing; thus, by targeting efforts on this subset, it should be possible eventually to eliminate chronic homelessness at a cost society can afford. The great majority of the homeless are only temporarily so, according to that study, and will be likely to emerge from it on their own (Gladwell 2006).

Thus, the awareness is growing that for both engagement and continuity of services, outreach services may provide crucial linkages between hospitals and clinics. If so, then this book may be appearing on the crest of a wave of events that could welcome its message. At least in New York, prison populations are declining significantly, as the unfairness of mandatory prison sentencing for minor drug offenses gains traction, particularly in the context of the economic burden of an annual cost of around $50,000 per inmate. Nationwide, public mental hospital systems have been slowly down-sizing, as state budgets, already strained, confront costs of up to $100,000 annually per institutionalized patient. Coincidentally, the need for new options has arisen in the context of a substantial diminution in state revenues, occasioned by the recession of 2007–2009. Thus, many individuals suffering either mental illness or substance abuse, or both, are being released to their home communities. Both private philanthropies, such as the George Soros Foundation and the Charles Koch Foundation, and policy-makers, including high-level elected officials, such as New York's governor, are publicizing and supporting new approaches to help these policies succeed.

Two more recent developments have the potential to stimulate the growth of outreach-and-engagement services, though it is still too early in both cases to tell how their positive impact will play out in the type of services that will emerge. The first of these is the Affordable Care Act itself, which promotes so-called Medical Homes and Accountable Care Organizations, both of which could incorporate ACT teams with "housing first" provisions into their overall structures. The second is a recently completed study indicating the potential for better outcomes for people with schizophrenia through what is likely to emerge quickly as a new "best practice." An extensive study led by Kane et al. (2015) involving multiple sites across the US produced such a dramatic result that it made the front page of the NY Times in mid-October. It found that the combination of modest medication and a range of supports that could be termed "psychotherapy" produced better outcomes for people with first-episode schizophrenia than did a focus on medication alone, usually in high doses, which had become the standard of care over the course of the previous three decades; furthermore, it found that the earlier this approach was initiated, the better the outcome. Psychiatrists in outreach settings should be among the first to have the opportunity to implement this finding (Section "Outreach Work Expands the Psychiatrist's Role").

My Personal Career Trajectory, Leading up to Outreach Psychiatry

Professionally, I was a late bloomer. I always knew I wanted to learn to talk to people who were considered out of their minds, but that was not enough to mark a career path. Toward the end of medical school, when I was applying to residency training programs in psychiatry, I came up against a training director whose question unsettled me. He asked me, reasonably enough, why I wanted to be a psychiatrist. After giving me a moment to mumble some platitudes about understanding and helping people, he interrupted with, "Yes, but what is your intellectual interest in psychiatry?" I had no answer, and the interview was over. Back in college I had been offered a personal introduction to Erik Erikson, who taught a course in the Human Life Cycle. I demurred, caught up in the neophyte illusion that it was better to avoid being influenced. I would not have known what to say to the great man at the time, but if I had accepted the invitation to meet him, I might have come away with some ideas that would have helped me answer the training director.

Fortunately, I landed a spot at another residency program, this one back at my own medical school. In my first year I treated patients from the local community who had been hospitalized for serious mental illnesses. I picked up the idea that it was possible to understand a system of care by learning "who was paying whom to do what for whom." And I learned from a social psychiatrist that there are some people who may find socialization itself unbearable. He provided an example from Cuba's experience: early on, people who were simply unable to adapt to routines and expectations were considered a sign of failure in the new social experiment, so they were rounded up from the streets and placed in institutions; unexpectedly, many died, in spite of adequate nutrition and reasonable care. But these random lessons did not coalesce into a direction for my future career.

The focus during my second year was on dynamic psychotherapy, also for hospitalized patients but, this time, selected for their teaching potential. Thanks to advice from a wise senior resident, I managed to get myself assigned to the premier preceptor for patients with schizophrenia, Harold Searles. Once a month he flew up from Washington, DC, to New York to teach a handful of us how to use our own inner responses to the patient, rather than the patient's words, to understand what s/he was trying to say. You might think that experience would have prepared me to answer other subsequent interviewers' questions, when I applied for a postgraduate research position at the National Institute for Mental Health, but you would be mistaken. So, my third and last year of residency was spent in a community psychiatry program in the South Bronx rather than in research in Bethesda. I enjoyed the setting, but the program was ahead of its time, so there was no large pool of graduating psychiatrists motivated to shed their white coats and wander the streets as we did. We were deprived even of the satisfaction of being trend-setters.

I even failed to mention to those interviewers at NIMH that I had had some exposure to research following my first year in medical school. I had landed on a research unit at Columbia that was investigating the effectiveness and safety of lithium carbonate, the first mood-stabilizer, for the treatment of bipolar disorder. Patients were referred to us from all over the country, sometimes with instructions from their employers to our investigators to help them settle down a bit, but not too much, since they were the creative force behind their respective companies. Once lithium received approval from the Food and Drug Administration as a first-line treatment, there was a credible story going around that, because differentiation from schizophrenia was so clouded, every patient at the Manhattan Psychiatric Center with a healthy heart and kidneys was given a trial of it. Many soon walked out the door, symptom-free and back in touch with reality after sometimes decades behind those walls.

After graduation from residency the question of military service came up. My application for discharge as a conscientious objector from the U.S. Army reserves, which I had entered under a government program, the Berry Plan, providing deferment for doctors completing their specialty training, forced me to define my role as a physician. I had known ever since entering medical school that my primary identification would be as a physician, and only secondarily, as a psychiatrist. I wrote that I defined my role as a physician as placing my medical knowledge at the disposal of my patients, so that they could make informed choices about their mental health treatments and life courses, something not compatible with the use of force. Somehow my definition satisfied the review board, who gave me the discharge. Alas, I was still unsure where to take it.

Once again, I moved back to a more generic path. I signed up for psychoanalytic training and was grateful to have the opportunity to matriculate at a classical institute for 8 years in the 1970s and to learn the value of close interaction with patients over an extended period—not to mention learning to take verbatim dictation, which was very useful in all my clinical work since, including the effort to gather the data necessary to write this book. I withdrew before completion of the program with the calculation, at least half-serious, that I might not live long enough to graduate. I considered the theory elegant and the training in listening closely to be invaluable, but psychoanalysis always seemed to me such a hermetic discipline, that I was glad to have the world of great fiction as a context for the purpose of validation.

During this time I also started a small private practice and became a teacher of psychiatric residents. People were very nice to me. I turned out to be pretty good at boiling a lot of disparate facts down to an acceptable generalization, so I asked questions of other people's presentations at departmental educational meetings. My successive department chairs apparently liked my questions, because they promoted me. My colleagues put up with me. My trainees were gracious enough to allow me my reductive generalizations. They even let me try out some of my fledgling ideas about how patients change (Section "My View of These Patients Change") in order to take charge of their symptoms and thus, of their lives.

I still did not have a specialty. Without one it is impossible to climb up the academic ladder in an academic department connected with a large university. I had written a few invited book reviews, but that was all. At parties I fielded the usual questions and jokes about psychiatrists. Some people were curious, though skeptical, to hear that "shrinks" actually derives historically from Freud's term *einschraenken* [literally, "to shrink into"], that is, to constrict one's focus, something he considered essential to understanding someone in depth—notwithstanding the mistaken but common assumption that it represents a shortened form of "head-shrinkers," a term used mockingly.

During those early years of professional practice, though still unsure where I was going to go with it, I had already formulated my theoretical orientation, one that was to change little over the ensuing years. Then as now, when a patient asked me about it, I would reply that I was a "Freudian," even knowing the historical baggage often associated with that designation. How could I have been otherwise, after eight rich years of training, even though I never finished? Usually that settled the matter. If the patient wanted to know what I meant, I would explain that, to me, it meant a commitment to paying close attention and trying continually to make sense of the whole picture without jumping to simplistic conclusions. It carried with it a belief in the importance of the unconscious mind, which is generally a lot wiser and more comprehensive than the conscious one, and likely to be several steps ahead of it, as well. Figuring out what it was saying might take a little practice but was no great feat. Dreams might turn out to be a help to the two of us, and there was no need to worry if you could not remember one right away: they would come along. The proof was in the result, anyway: either problems got solved or they did not. Proving the theory was beside the point. The rest seemed like details or footnotes.

Declining the invitation to meet Erikson while in college showed that I had not realized the importance of attaching myself to someone who represented a model of what I wanted to become. Working for and with such a person would have presented the opportunity, much earlier on, to learn what s/he had figured out about putting theory and practice together. Apparently I had something in common with a patient of mine during those early years of practice. While still a young woman, she had shown considerable promise as a dancer and had been accepted into Martha Graham's company. But then her career came to an abrupt halt. You will understand why Graham's words to her have stuck with me. "Your problem," she said to my patient, "is that you will never submit!" Like my patient I needed to follow the trail that a truly creative person had already blazed, if I was to avoid getting lost, myself.

In retrospect it is fairly obvious where I had to look. Just as Willie Sutton had figured out that he had to rob banks, if his goal was to find the money, so I should have figured out that I had to go into the public mental health system, where people with serious mental illnesses wind up getting treated, if my goal was to understand more about those illnesses. That is the other place for a psychiatrist to go to go if he has missed the chance to go into research. But getting there took me almost another two decades.

Finally, as the saying goes, "things happened." With very little effort on my part, I wound up with a responsible position in the organization best suited to my main professional interest and with the mentor and supervisor who was to show me how to develop it into something definable at last. As far as I was concerned, there was no turning back. At last, in my early 50s and halfway through my professional career, I had been given yet another chance, and I was not going to let it slip away again. My mentor/supervisor, John Oldham, was from the start and continued to the end to be more of a model than I could have wished for, and attaching myself to him did not feel one bit like submitting.

Things started out slowly enough: at NYS-OMH, where I landed the job, I was assigned to oversee the distribution of the agency's funding support for psychiatric residents at university-based training programs around the state, with the goal of promoting their exposure to public-sector patients, especially those confined to state-run psychiatric facilities. The knowledge base for that assignment was familiar enough to me, because I had been a residency training director myself and also had had plenty of in-hospital experience treating patients.

Then things began to accelerate. I had not reckoned on the push I was about to receive from a dynamic commissioner who was determined to put into practice his notion of recovery from serious mental illness. This notion challenged the received knowledge of just about everyone in his agency. There was plenty of resistance to recalibrating goals beyond symptom control. I thought he sounded good in theory but vague in implementation, and he had heard a rumor that I was one of those traditional psychiatrists more protective of our own turf than committed to helping patients move on with their goals. The Commissioner reported directly to the state's Deputy Secretary for Human Services, whom the governor respected highly, and the Secretary felt the same way about the Commissioner, so there was no question as to whose attitude would prevail. Both he and I, fortunately for me, came to know each other better, though there were some rough spots along the way. Indeed, without Oldham's continual protection, my exposure might have ended prematurely on more than one occasion.

I learned many things about how a large bureaucracy can move toward successful change. One is that it takes a high-level administrator who grasps the need to allow for some flexibility when implementing new policies. I had been fortunate enough to encounter someone like this, namely, NYS-OMH's Chief Operating Officer. Even though the state-run clinics had been scheduled to close, he accepted my plea to preserve an essential training experience at one of them, because without this experience the residency program would have lost accreditation. But such administrators are rare.

I am a clinician at heart, and we clinicians get our initial bearings by examining individual patients, rather than by trying to figure out the larger systems we are working in. So, I set about attending to my various administrative duties by making myself available to my psychiatric colleagues throughout NYS-OMH's hospitals as a case-consultant. Whenever they invited me for a consultation, I figured I could take the opportunity to inquire of the local psychiatrists how much teaching they were doing, and how the residents assigned to them were going about learning public psychiatry. Meanwhile, I could get to know the system by getting to know how the individual patients were being treated.

Early on, I got lucky with a particularly challenging one. The staff psychiatrists had diagnosed him as having schizophrenia, on the basis of his cardinal symptom of pica, that is, repeatedly ingesting non-food items—in his case, bits of Styrofoam, paper clips, and scissors, many of which had to be removed surgically. They had tried unsuccessfully to stop him by forcing him to wear a thick, plastic mask for increasing periods of time, noting how long those periods subsequently prevented the emergence of his symptom—something right out of Dumas' *Man in the Iron Mask*. But it remained a losing battle. Now they were hopeful that with my administrative connections, I might be able to access a then-new medication for him, clozapine, uniquely effective for nonresponsive schizophrenia. However, I had never heard that pica was a symptom of schizophrenia; rather, it is associated with a genetic disorder or in some cases a vitamin deficiency and usually shows up in young children as transient eating of dirt. Furthermore, the staff psychiatrists did not report the patient as having any of the symptoms that are characteristic of schizophrenia.

So, even before consulting on the patient, I was thinking about an organic condition. The clinical staff brought him out and enumerated the many instances of his single sign of disturbed behavior. When I got to interview him, the first thing he said to me was, "Doc, I promise I'll never pick up and eat any of those things again." My hunch was confirmed by a simple, brief neurological test I remembered from medical school, which suggested that he had a neurological problem, though I was not sure this was clear to the many clinical staff who were in attendance. What I restrained myself from saying was that I had the impulse to drive my car over the mask they had had fashioned at great expense, with the best of intentions, to "de-condition" him, lest they ever consider using it on him again. After my consultation I sought out a neurosurgeon who had been one of my teachers back in medical school, who requested a CAT scan using a contrast medium for the purpose of diagnosis, adding that he wanted the films themselves, rather than a report of what they showed. Getting them took several months, as it happened, but the result was more than worth the effort. I can still remember his calling me into his office, moments after I hand-delivered them. He assumed even I would have no trouble noticing the Christmas-tree-light-bulb-sized tumor that fairly glowed white against the gray-and-black film.

But the preparations were still far from over. I was informed by the treating psychiatrist that because of his schizophrenia the patient was deemed incompetent to provide his consent for surgery, so that, if I wanted to proceed, I would need to return to the hospital where he resided and obtain it myself; this I duly did. "Doc," the patient asked, "could I die from this operation?" "It is highly unlikely," I replied, "but the answer to your question is certainly 'yes.'" "Doc, would you have this operation?" was his next question. "Absolutely," I replied with conviction, "because I think it will be successful in helping you to stop eating those things, and I also believe that the consequences of not having it are likely to be much worse." He signed the form. Next, I was called in by NYS-OMH's chief counsel, who admonished me that, if there were any untoward result from this operation, my career would be over, and asked whether I might like to reconsider. I accepted his terms. The expected outcome ensued: in an 8-h procedure, the surgeon successfully removed the man's benign teratoma, a tumor that had been pressing down on his hypothalamus, the part of the brain that controls appetite and presumably, thereby, had been causing his strange behavior. If left untreated, it also would likely have led to his demise. My reputation got a big boost.

Finding what used to be called an "organic" basis for this man's presumably schizophrenic behavior so early in my tenure with NYS-OMH was fortuitous. I have certainly been guilty of confusing the two, more than once, in the long course of my clinical career. But it is at least consistent with my conviction, shared by virtually all general medical specialists, that diagnosis matters, because it combines both past history and present symptoms in order to try to predict what is likely to happen in the future. However, I have encountered many psychiatrists who do not share this view. Instead, they concentrate on symptoms of disturbed behavior with the goal of suppressing them, whatever their origin, and further, if they succeed, attribute the improvement to the effects of their intervention. Then they proceed to infer a diagnosis from the result, retrospectively, almost as an afterthought, useful for record-keeping purposes.

Concurrent with my position at NYS-OMH, this combined interest landed me a gratifying role at a community hospital for two decades as a preceptor in bedside clinical interviewing to medical students learning internal medicine. On the wall of our conference room was a plaque featuring a dictum by William Osler, who introduced bedside teaching. It read, "To treat a patient it is not enough to understand him or even the world in which he lives: we must also understand his position in that world." You can imagine that these words were like music to my ears. By the end of my tenure there, the role I was allowed to play, as a "consultation-liaison psychiatrist," was beginning to expand into a potentially larger role as part of a new model of treatment in which psychiatry and general medicine are combined, now known as "integrated care."

What drew me to clinical medicine in the first place, and what I have continued to enjoy about it ever since, is that there is something "real" that happens "out there" with the patient, and not merely in the mind of the practitioner. Mostly, we are trying out this and that, however much we aim to apply scientific knowledge to defined conditions. Practice guidelines help, but they are not dispositive, because real-world conditions vary, and because patient responses to the same treatments vary to such a daunting degree. But what happens is not simply a matter of opinion: the patients get better, or they do not. Furthermore, they have a real say in the matter, and they express this by voting with their feet: if they like what is happening, they come back for more; otherwise, they do not, provided that they have a choice.

To finish this story, I would have to acknowledge that never, in the dozen or so years thereafter, in all the consultations I was invited to perform around the far reaches of the Empire State, was I to be so dramatically successful again in demonstrating the connection between body and mind. However, through these encounters, I did begin gradually to formulate my own impressions of what the state psychiatric hospital system was aimed at achieving. It served as the back-up system for all the community hospital psychiatric in-patient units, receiving all the patients who did not manage to get control over their disruptive or self-destructive behavior after a short period of time, usually defined as 1–2 months. This aim makes a certain amount of sense; however, there was a big problem at the "back end": because of a lack of effective follow-up available to patients who have spent long periods in state hospitals, they remained vulnerable to early and frequent returns; furthermore, they tended to develop dependency on structured support, and they missed out on the life experiences that might have taught them better than any of us clinicians could, to manage their own symptoms in the service of moving on toward their own goals.

A manifestation of this skewed process was that patients frequently manifested a recurrence, in the days just prior to discharge, of symptoms that had brought them to the psychiatric hospitals in the first place. Was this a sign that they needed further treatment, via an extension of their stay, or was it predominantly an indication of the anxiety they faced over the prospect of independence, after a long period without it? Searles had taught us that what we needed to do was to identify with both sides of the patients' intense ambivalence about discharge, so that they could move on beyond the anxiety that it typically aroused.

For example, I interviewed a 22-year-old woman, hospitalized since age 16 for symptoms of "psychosis," whose initial manifestation had been limited to a hallucination of her closest girlfriend, standing at night at the edge of her bed. This girlfriend had been struck and killed by a car, precipitating the patient's hospitalization. Whenever she appeared ready for discharge, she would become intensely anxious, and her symptom would return. Even setting aside the question of the validity of a diagnosis of schizophrenia for this single symptom, I would find it hard to justify 6 years' hospitalization on the basis that her symptom would return just prior to each proposed discharge date.

Another woman I interviewed was in her 40s. She had long been detained because of intermittent suicide threats over a period of several years. She explained to me that she had made specific plans with a fellow-patient to set up a household and to work for a community agency that provided services to children. Furthermore, she continued, as far as her risk of suicide went, she could carry it out at any time, whether confined to the hospital or not, and that it should play no adverse role in the decision regarding her discharge. Despite my efforts, the staff in both cases concluded that longer stays were needed; such was the prevalent thinking. They might not have believed Searles, either, if he had tried to explain that her ambivalence about leaving did not simply mean that she opposed it. My explanation, tacked onto his, would have added that her symptom resulted from the anxiety of reentering a world she had left behind so much earlier.

NYS-OMH continued to "talk the talk" of recovery and of patients' setting their own priorities, but the structure for "walking the walk" to implement such a change remained elusive. Many of us hoped it might at last materialize, when the Community Reinvestment Act was signed in 1994 by every member of the state legislature and celebrated with great fanfare by the governor and my Commissioner at Fountain House. Hopes arose that, under this legislation, several state psychiatric hospitals would be closed and the savings reinvested in community mental health services. A few closings did result, but little reinvestment followed.

For my last 2 years with NYS-OMH, after Oldham moved on, I took his place as Chief Medical Officer (acting). I managed to introduce a few projects appropriate to that role. One was aimed at reducing the incidence of prescribing multiple antipsychotics to the same patient, a practice that has repeatedly been shown to add side effects without measureable benefit. The lead-up to implementing the reduction involved a realization among in-patient psychiatrists that the doses they prescribed were unsustainable in community settings, while psychiatrists in those settings feared to reduce them, lest they be blamed for any relapses. In response a few of our state hospitals managed to reduce the incidence of this practice significantly.

Another project was to give a presentation to my fellow state medical directors about the possible cause of the of excess premature mortality, also called the "longevity gap," long observed but inadequately understood, whereby people with serious mental illness died decades younger than their peers. My chief internist had observed that the elderly patients in our state hospitals did not die early, as they would have been expected to do, if they had been living in the community. He wondered whether the difference in their fate might result from their regularly receiving good general medical care for the usual chronic conditions that cause deaths in the general population, namely, hypertension, diabetes, and cardiovascular disease. In the community such patients do not receive the necessary care, presumably due to the mutual fear of the patients and their physicians. Unfortunately, many psychiatrists share this fear—and thus, avoidance—with their non-psychiatric medical colleagues.

Also, I continued to consult on challenging patients across the state. Most of them, though certainly not all, seemed to me to have gotten pretty much what they could from their hospital stays, and many of them indicated that they were ready to move on; however, my efforts to push my 800 psychiatrist-colleagues at NYS-OMH to try lowering medications, supporting their patients' spontaneous efforts at independence, and above all, releasing them sooner rather than later from our institutions into the community, were not generally welcomed: there always seemed to be one more behavioral symptom that got in the way. I would have to grant that my last exposure to community psychiatry had been decades earlier; thus, my personal bias toward supporting patient autonomy rather than practicing paternalism—an extension of what I had told the Armed Services review board—remained no more than a bias. I could not speak convincingly about how it would play out in practice. In my experience people do not change their behavior because you have presented them with a new theory; rather, what carries conviction is that tone in your voice that comes from having tried something that seemed to work out, yourself.

But I walked away from NYS-OMH a happy man: for nearly a decade and a half, I had worked in the public sector to try to improve services for the people with the conditions that had brought me into the field of medicine in the first place. These had expanded well beyond schizophrenia and bipolar illness to include, as noted above, post-traumatic disorders, substance abuse, and childhood disorders, and familiarity with both civil and forensic institutional settings. I no longer had any doubt as to who I was: a public psychiatrist.

The question I still needed to answer for myself was whether people released from hospitals or brought in from the streets could indeed figure out how to manage their symptoms and get on with their lives, if given acceptable housing and ongoing support. I had heard about outreach services for those not yet settled in. Were those services the answer? So, I abandoned my fond hopes of retirement at 64 and jumped at an offer to work for an agency that was dedicated to addressing that question. Now I would have the chance to see how my notions of recovery, where the patient is the "locus of care," played out in the real world. There was a considerable challenge in taking this step: how well would I do at implementing the kinds of practices I had urged my fellow NYS-OMH psychiatrists to follow? My position with the next agency provided me with the experience that this book is about. For starters, it got me back into working as a front-line provider of services to people with serious mental illness, rather than as a teacher, administrator, or consultant.

The Pathways Model

In the spring of 2005 I took a position as the psychiatrist on an outreach team based in Jamaica, Queens, and administered by a private, not-for-profit agency. It received patients through public referral agencies, including state mental hospitals, mental health courts, and later on, prisons. I had heard about this agency during my tenure at NYS-OMH and been introduced to its founder and director by a noted social scientist we both admired, so it was not entirely a leap into the unknown.

Pathways to Housing was founded in 1992 to provide community outreach services to people suffering serious mental illness with or without addiction, who were homeless. It was the creation of a psychologist, Sam Tsemberis, out of two essential ingredients. The first of these was "housing first," and the second, ACT services.

The first of these means that we do not wait for clients to "earn" admission to housing by meeting particular standards of behavior, but instead, give it to them from the start and then proceed to do what we can to keep them in it, as safe from harm and as tolerable to their neighbors, building superintendents, and landlords as possible. Having a roof over one's head means more than having a safe place to go to or an address to give the pharmacist when a prescription refill is due; it also means an address where one can be located for follow-up or for accompaniment to one's primary-care physician. These were market-rate apartments or, in some instances, houses that Pathways was able to purchase, thanks to a donation, at the time of the agency's inception. That is, none were group homes and none came with a live-in staff member. All were located in working-class neighborhoods in Jamaica, Queens.

The second of these ingredients, ACT services, refers to a model for providing outreach—or, more properly, outreach-plus-engagement, the latter being the purpose of outreach in the first place; the relationship between the two is a bit like that between stability and recovery: you cannot have one without the other. ACT was developed in the mid-70s by Stein, Test, and their colleagues in Madison, Wisconsin (Section "What is Recovery, and How Does it Relate to Stability?"). This model describes a team of clinicians who provide social support, psychiatric treatment, and advocacy. Team members include specialists in substance abuse, family therapy, and employment counseling, along with the usual psychiatrist, nurse, and social worker. ACT differs from traditional clinic services, in that it reaches out to and actively engages patients where they live, rather than waiting for them to show up at agency offices.

In contrast to in-patient teams ACT teams hold few administrative meetings; instead, team members mostly communicate informally while providing direct services in community settings. In contrast to case-management the teams themselves provide the services, rather than merely brokering or overseeing them. In recent times there has also been a growing effort to include on such teams a so-called "peer-specialist," meaning, a former patient who has graduated to the role of service-provider and has received training and certification, sometimes in one of the aforementioned professional roles. Though the appreciation of the benefits of employing peers in a range of clinical roles is only recently coming in for attention, it is not a new role. More than 40 years ago Robert Lifton came to believe that the most capable and credible clinicians for traumatized Viet Nam War veterans were their battlefield-tested peers, further armed with some clinical training (Lifton 1973).

More important than professional background is the range of personalities, each contributing an individual perspective, based on her/his own life experience, which helps round out the picture of each patient to enhance understanding and promote empathy; furthermore, the team members support each other, not only emotionally but also literally, in the provision of services, as will be illustrated in several of the succeeding chapters (Chaps. 2, 4, 6, 8).

ACT's effectiveness has been repeatedly and strongly validated by research over the decades since; however, it was never integrated into standard residency training outside of public psychiatry fellowships, of which only a handful exist, even now. Therefore, most psychiatrists know it only in theory or by hearsay—I certainly did not, prior to this experience, and few would credit it with providing an essential link in the continuity of care for a distinct population.

The essence of outreach services is the home visit. It would be difficult to overstate the value of such a visit, in terms of understanding how that woman or man is managing her/his own life, both in real time and over time. One glance— sometimes it's a whiff—at the order or disorder, cheerfulness or drabness, taste or clutter, tells me more than a half-year of weekly visits to my private office, where I have maintained a practice in psychotherapy and pharmacotherapy for over 40 years. There I remain continually chagrinned at which obvious element in the patient's environment or habits I have failed to inquire about or even to realize. And that is even before I get a look into the refrigerator and food shelves, to see whether they contain cereals, fresh fruits and vegetables, and healthy beverages—or junk food and sugared drinks.

You might suppose that privacy considerations would interfere here; after all, in my private practice, I have never entered patients' homes except for rare visits to home-bound geriatric patients. But, as in so many situations, the reality presents fewer obstacles than the theory would predict: in my 6 years at Pathways, I was never refused entry into a patient's home. It is the sense of working on the problems together that prevails.

As for privacy in my own Pathways office, there was none. It had four thin walls and a door, but they presented only visual, not auditory privacy. As if to make the point, the space was open at the top, not reaching the ceiling of the room. That allowed for good air circulation, which was a boon during warmer months but less so during colder ones. No one seemed to mind. A few colored paintings and pencil drawings adorned my walls, but these were meaningful mostly to those who had produced them, and I was initially unaware of who had done so. Some patients occasionally brought me their drawings from art group, which I would add to what was already there, if space permitted. Some scarred, torn linoleum may have covered the floor, but no amount of mopping with ammonia could make it shine. And something else about the general setting: we had a receptionist with excellent interpersonal skills, who was an important member of our team, but she was so busy taking care of clients' financial issues, including paying their monthly bills, that she had no time to manage my schedule or any other staff member's. I made one up and gave her a copy, so she would know whom to expect each day. I will come back to her at one sad point in my last chapter (Section "Risks of Physical Harm to Outreach Clinicians"). This was definitely a do-it-yourself operation.

Next in order of importance for places where we catch up with patients is the whole range of healthcare settings, from hospitals to emergency rooms to general medical clinics. Here, too, it would be hard to overstate the impact, in terms of efficiency of services, of meeting up with patients in these settings. So much did the medical staff welcome my being able to provide clinical information as to why our patients required their services at those times, and my demonstration of readiness to help them return home as soon as possible, that they routinely bumped them to the head of the emergency room triage lines. Furthermore, getting to know medical and nursing staff in these settings personally meant a promise of future collaborations; indeed, it seemed that many of those clinicians, either immediately or gradually, without formal invitation, became extensions of my team, building relationships that helped manage not only the patients of immediate and ongoing concern, but also those whom we were to encounter together in the future. I became a familiar presence, not only in the half-dozen local hospitals in Queens, but also in some similar facilities in The Bronx, Manhattan, Brooklyn, Westchester, and beyond, where our patients frequently showed up for evaluation and treatment.

It took a few months to establish my role on my own Pathways team. I never met my predecessor, but the role that person established must have involved hospitalizing the patients considerably more frequently than I was used to or thought necessary. That much I deduced from noting how many of my patients were being hospitalized during the five days of the week that I was not scheduled. (note: Pathways refers to the people it cares for as its clients; because I am a doctor, I refer to those I treat as my patients, even though I am aware that, for historical reasons, "my patients" will sound paternalistic to some of you.) My team members were, understandably, skeptical about the infrequency of my resort to hospitalization. For the first few months my Wednesday arrivals typically began with visits to the local hospitals to which team members had sent them, invariably describing them as having "relapsed." They may have been even more dubious when it became apparent that, once there, I had proceeded to interview the patient and speak with her/his psychiatrist, arrange for release, and take her/him home. Gradually, the team must have gotten sufficiently used to my view, or my persistence, that they gave this up. Instead, they presented their concerns to me during my two regular work days. During my 6 years several of my patients presented themselves for hospitalization on days when I was not available, and I am sure I must have asked on a given occasion whether one of them had felt it might be necessary (Section "Risks of Physical Harm to Outreach Clinicians"), but I cannot recall ever having encouraged any of them to do so.

As far as feeling I belonged on the team, that began three months into my tenure, when our peer-specialist, who was also the team's substance abuse counselor, told me, late one afternoon, as I was leaving, "You are making a real difference here."

From that moment on I felt I had arrived. You will learn more about him in several of the narratives below (Chaps. 2, 4).

The bottom line is that we showed up wherever our patients needed us to. I went grocery shopping with some, met others outside the door of their temporary-work sites, accompanied others to colleges where one hoped to rematriculate and another, to take prep classes for his high school equivalency exam. On a couple of occasions I spent most of a day at the local Medicaid office, trying to facilitate their getting back onto the rolls, from which so many were routinely stricken for failure to renew eligibility—a common problem for people who have trouble getting into their mailboxes or reading forms. Supervisors at those offices expressed surprise at my showing up there with their clients but, in response, they regularly expedited the process for me.

Right now, you may be wondering about a couple of things: first, how does a psychiatrist have the time to spend on all these apparently non-medical pursuits; and second, what was the tab for all these services? So, let me give you some idea of the parameters. I was paid for eight hours per day, two days per week, to treat 30 of my own patients and to consult on another 30, who were treated by our psychiatric nurse practitioner (PNP). I was responsible for entering a note describing each patient encounter by the close of business each day. Sometimes this required putting in an extra unpaid hour, but it was just as well that way, because it meant I did not have to take my work home with me—until this past year, when I began writing this book! Over the 6 years of employment I averaged five notes per day, a number that may seem luxurious to some of you practitioners; however, given the amount of time outreach work takes in transit, there was scarcely ever a free moment. You can imagine I was getting plenty of exercise going from place to place.

My agency was funded by capitated Medicaid payments of $1500 per month per patient, which their covered ACT services, including mental health. Fee-for-Service Medicaid covered their general health services. Two-thirds of their monthly rent came from city, state, and federal housing contracts; the other third came out of their monthly SSI allotment. Tacitly and overtly, my agency recognized that the only way we were going to promote autonomy for our clients was to give us some of the same, including the frequency and location of our encounters. Therefore, we were given a lot of freedom and encouraged to be creative and flexible. So, you might just as well ask the converse of those things you were wondering about: how else than by accompanying our patients on their daily rounds were we going to figure out how they were managing and what help they wanted?

One more thing about the creativity and flexibility I just mentioned: there is a theory behind this approach, called "motivational interviewing." I have not looked into it further than a general understanding, but what I take it to mean is that the psychiatrist has absolutely no goal for her-/himself in the interview, other than to help the patient figure out her/his own goals. That includes, as an extreme example, foregoing even the goal of encouraging a substance-abusing person give up those substances. This perspective is not only difficult for most traditional medical types like me to achieve; it is also difficult for our patients to believe we have it in mind.

They are long accustomed to being told by professionals what they need to do. So, it takes time to develop the particular kind of relationship Pathways was encouraging—from months to a couple of years. But then, things would begin to happen.

You may share my skepticism of newer and not-quite-proven trends that are also counterintuitive from some perspectives. If so, let me refer you to something written over 50 years ago by my first distinguished preceptor, Harold Searles (Section "Why We Need Expanded Outreach Services"), about the perspective he thought was crucial for doing psychoanalytic therapy with people with schizophrenia (Searles 1961): "One leaves in the patient's hands the choice as to whether he wants to spend the rest of his life in a mental hospital, or whether he wants, instead, to become well. These are no mere words, but the expression of a deep and genuine feeling-orientation." Does this not sound to you like an elegant, early formulation of motivational interviewing? It certainly does to me.

Pathways' treatment philosophy came down firmly on the side of what today has in many circles become a slogan, "shared decision-making," which welcomes a variety of voices and perspectives, underwrites patient autonomy, and affirms continuity between disabling and extreme states of experience and those more common in everyday life. You will imagine by now that I did not need much convincing.

Goal-setting, in my experience, proceeds differently with each patient. There are a number of obvious reasons why simply inquiring after them is not terribly productive. First, many of us, patients or not, just do not know what they are; if we do, as some of the patients described later will demonstrate, we have not felt free to pursue them, whether out of our own doubts or because someone else has discouraged us. Second, in typical clinician-patient encounters, where symptoms and treatments are the stock-in-trade, patients become so accustomed to being prescribed treatments, with which they are expected to be compliant, that such an inquiry seems, at best, insincere, and at worst, a first step toward establishing leverage over them. Third, some material goals, such as the need for shelter, food, and access to transportation, are so universal that may seem obvious or banal. So, it seems to me that the best course is to wait for trust to develop and, meanwhile, keep one's ears and eyes open for hints of the patient's priorities.

Do you want to object at this point that many of those goals would be unrealistic? If so, you will have to read on, to some of the narratives themselves. Then you can judge for yourself.

Let me elaborate for a moment on our policy toward substance abuse, which has increasingly wide currency under the name of "harm-reduction." This policy means accepting substance use and even abuse, unless or until the patient decides to discontinue it. In the interim we attempt to limit its harmful consequences, among them, the risk of exposure to serious infection, and to support clients' efforts to reduce intake. It avoids an obvious pitfall of the policy in effect almost universally during my early years of training and practice, which was to forbid all substance abuse as a condition of psychiatric treatment. This old policy precluded a large proportion of patients with mental illnesses from receiving psychiatric treatment at all. The new one provided time for a therapeutic relationship to develop. It accorded with the underlying principle of the clinician's having no fixed agenda other than helping the patient identify and pursue hers/his. However, when the substance abuse presents an increasing threat to life or health, it tests the clinician's commitment to this policy—not that there is any viable alternative: exhortations do not work very often, and the moment rarely arrives at which the threat can be considered so imminent as to trigger an involuntary hospitalization.

Pathways exuded self-confidence for what it could offer and set the model for the kind of flexibility and creativity needed for its success. For help with particularly challenging situations, both clinical and administrative, as you will read below (Chaps. 2, 9), I turned to our clinical director, Sheryl Silver. Its foundation seemed so solid.

But in fact it was subject, like any real-world institution, to a changing political and historical environment. Four years into my tenure there, it came under new pressure. Some of the same thoughtful policy-makers who had approved it for Medicaid funding in the first place began to wonder whether, if such a modest level of investment could stabilize a small cohort of previously problematic patients, why could it not be scaled up to accommodate much larger and other types of cohorts, such as families or parolees? Pathways would have been delighted either to expand its scope or to help train other agencies. The only problem was that the bureaucracies seeking to expand our existing capacity did not intend to offer increased funding; instead, they suggested that we might create the needed capacity ourselves, by discharging clients who had been with us for a specified period of time. It mattered little to them that the ACT model which guided our approach included an open-ended commitment to our clients, or that very little research literature suggested that they would be able to find permanent housing on their own without our guarantee to prospective landlords of financial backing. This pressure resulted in a policy of discharging clients to other agencies that provided supported housing services alone, without ACT services, after a ceremony which we euphemistically referred to as "graduation." This policy significantly affected—though not always for the worse— the trajectories of several of the patients whose narratives you will find below.

As for the safety of clinicians practicing in this setting, the proof, once again, was in the process, rather than in a priori concerns. On the street we were mostly protected by our reputation as clinicians with no connection to the civil authorities, who, therefore, presented no threat to some neighborhood figures with whom our clients dealt, such as drug-dealers. We were not looking for trouble, so trouble was not directed our way. This was something I had learned three decades earlier, during my first community psychiatry experience, walking the streets of the South Bronx (Section "My Personal Career Trajectory, Leading up to Outreach Psychiatry"). When one has a legitimate purpose in a neighborhood and acts as if that is the only reason for being there, the locals somehow get the message.

It should be clear by now that this whole experience was much more than an opportunity to provide care and treatment. I was determined, for my own reasons, to find out whether people burdened with these awful conditions could get back onto —or get onto, for the first time—the track they had in mind for themselves. It should not come as a surprise if it turned out that what they needed in order to accomplish this was just the same kind of encouragement that the rest of us needed and received during the course of our own development.

I believed from first-hand experience that my Pathways patients were, at the point that they came to us, just as ill as were the people confined in my state's mental hospitals, and that they were not yet stable enough to manage for themselves. So for me the stakes in answering these questions were almost as high as they were for our patients and for all the others who might stand in their shoes, and for the system as a whole. The community was watching, and it had its own concerns about both safety and unsightliness. What kept me going, therefore, were the intellectual and emotional satisfactions of figuring out, from personal observation and experience, just how the process would unfold. Taking charge of one's illness is a process, not an event; therefore, unless the patient is the driver, change will be transient at best. The warm welcome and generosity of my patients were icing on the cake.

My View of How These Patients Change

My personal framework for posing these questions was based on the potential each of us has for change. Some years ago I wrote a book (Tucker 2007) about how writers of literary short stories describe how fictional characters change at different stages of the life cycle. As a framework for describing ongoing development throughout life I used the eight such stages in Erikson's schema—yes, Erikson at last! These writers have illustrated how it comes about and have even suggested what it may mean in the future lives of their fictional characters. I have hosted a workshop for mental health professionals for the past decade to discuss how change looks in these short stories and to consider how to use them in our teaching and practice. But is change the same thing for these very ill patients? Would they define their problems as their fellow citizens might, who consider them a nuisance, a burden, or a threat? Do these patients even want to change? If so, what would they have to do for themselves to make it happen? And not incidentally, what could we professionals do to support them, if they did?

Change does not mean cure, any more than it does with chronic general medical illnesses, such as diabetes, hypertension, and asthma, which also have strong genetic components; however it does fit nicely into the concept of recovery, which the advocacy movement has been promoting for three decades, and it coincides nicely with the emergence of the evidence from systematic research. I would say that the essence of change for the patients who shared their lives with me over the ensuing 6 years was that they managed to find a way to take charge of their illnesses through taking charge of their own lives, rather than submitting to the fate that those illnesses—and treatment-as-usual—was imposing on them. No more than half of those I got to know well managed to do this, and each of their stories was quite distinct and personal. It did not revolve around any of the four measures of stability that I described at the beginning (Section "What is Recovery, and How Does it

Relate to Stability?"), because, not surprisingly, those measures were only of secondary interest to them. What they cared about, explicitly, or, more commonly, implicitly, was a personal goal: something that s/he wanted to bring about, just as people without serious mental illnesses do. That is, the change each patient underwent was a manifestation of each one's recovery.

From this perspective the management of their illnesses and thus, their achievement of stability, was merely a by-product. Examples included maintaining one's apartment to preserve the desired security and privacy; being accorded a deserved measure of respect or recognition; expressing a genuine commitment to another person, perhaps long known but not fully appreciated; having one's wishes for independence validated; having one's core identity affirmed; finding an activity so enjoyable as to make it worth staying out of trouble; proving to some person in authority that s/he had underestimated her/him; accepting limited but predictable satisfactions rather than grand but risky ones; resisting distractions; or finding a personal narrative that made sense out of confusing failures that were not, given the combination of one's genetic liabilities, life experiences, and society's pessimism, entirely one's own fault.

It seems to me that health issues are usually not and should not be anyone's central preoccupation, outside a situation of acute pain, injury, or illness, or the threat of death or bodily harm. This would certainly apply also to people with serious mental illness. Invoking John Nash (Section "What is Recovery, and How Does it Relate to Stability?") again, I would say that their central preoccupations are their life goals. In this view the role of the psychiatrist or other mental health clinician is to help them proceed toward achieving them, and if that is happening, then they will take care of the illness, almost incidentally. This remains true, even in the face of occasional, brief relapses, which therefore do not, in themselves, imply failure.

The psychiatrist's role as a change agent in promoting recovery appears in various guises in the world's collection of literary short stories, most of which include the ideal or the most likely or perhaps even the only possible change agent. I asked myself over and over what the relationship was between my role and the patients' choices to move forward with their lives. I provided diagnoses, often either modified or greatly altered from previous ones given to them. I provided a forum for trials of medications that we discussed and evaluated together. I advocated on their behalf with providers of general health services. I assuaged family members' concerns, when I could. I mediated with courts and parole officers. I attended to a host of more mundane matters, such as assessing and ameliorating, if possible, the condition of their apartments, sometimes even by interceding with their landlords, who were receptive because our policy of guaranteeing the rents was reassuring to them, and who usually met us halfway.

Overall, my role boiled down to being an observer and a source of information, to be accessed if and when they asked for it. Again and again, they did: they let me into their lives and shared them with me. The changes which these personal motives precipitated were only changes in process, for, as in short stories, the outcomes remain in the future. Six years represent only a cross-sectional segment of someone's life. In the end what kept coming back to me was the idea that I was simply trying to hold onto their coattails long enough, while they decided how they wanted to use me to pursue their available options.

Maybe this is the place to jump ahead a little and anticipate a question that may come to you when you get to the narratives, namely, whether my theoretical orientation, noted above (Section "Why We Need Expanded Outreach Services"), had to be modified here from what it was with my private patients. There are two issues at play here with every patient, over time: the urgency of the current problem, and psychological-mindedness, also called "insight." As for the latter, I find that it is in short supply with most people, myself included. Other than a few flashes of it, I did not begin to acquire even a modest amount of it until quite recently in the course of my 40 + years of dynamic psychotherapy; to my knowledge, the only person who publicly admitted to having even more years of such therapy was the late Oliver Sacks.

As for the former, there is no question but that my Pathways patients faced more environmental stressors, starting with recent homelessness, than did my private patients, whose stressors were more likely interpersonal ones. But then, I had more resources at my disposal, starting with my fellow team members and continuing through a range of agencies. I was in the habit of calling for help from other professionals for both groups of patients. As for my guesses about the unspoken motivations Gary had for dressing up (Chap. 2), or Alex for some of his erratic behavior (Chap. 8), or Seema for her intense attachment to me (Chap. 12)—those may tell you more about me than about them: I do not customarily go in much for those kinds of explanations, except when they may help alleviate someone's guilt or despair, or otherwise help them keep focused on their goals. As for distortions in their view of me that come from their assessment of powerful figures in their past, I do not customarily worry about those either, as long as they are positive, whether deservedly or not: rather, I bring them up only if they are negative and getting in our way.

When nothing else works, and I am becoming desperate, I resort to bringing a literary short story into the treatment setting, in order to give us both a moment of reprieve and a gratifying focus from which to restart our approaches to the problem at hand. Team members suggested several times that I consider convening a short story workshop for my Pathways patients. Alas, I did not manage to find a reliably free hour a week to schedule this, so I was able to try it out only with one patient (Chap. 4); from the result I wish in retrospect I had tried harder.

How These Narratives Emerged

Narrative medicine has been around for decades. I am familiar with at least two widely practiced versions, both of them formulated and disseminated widely, long before I sat down to write. In the 1980s Donald Spence and Roy Shafer introduced one of them, the idea that the construction of a narrative was central to the process of psychoanalysis. The goal was to develop one that integrated the events of the patient's past and present life into a serviceable form that the patient could embrace and use to expand her/his current life choices. More recently, Columbia's Rita Charon updated that earlier version and applied it to narratives explicitly written by patients or healthcare professionals, including students, about their experiences with illness and healing.

In addition she drew on her wide familiarity with fictional literature to introduce a second version, which promoted the study of particular works of great literature as a way to enhance physicians' ability to empathize with their patients. She established a division of narrative medicine within Columbia's Department of Medicine that included both versions. This second approach is elsewhere known as medical humanities, a version of which I tried to illustrate in my earlier book.

The narratives here represent my attempt at the former version, with the particular aim of showing how people learn from a series of experiences to solve a practical problem they have set for themselves. This learning happens to occur in the context of a therapeutic relationship, but that is not the only, or even the principal context of learning: life, after all, is the great teacher. My examples assume that the patients do not necessarily know what problem has the highest priority when things begin, and that the psychiatrist certainly does not know it. Gradually, it becomes clear to both of us, and sometimes, the patient solves it. I hope I can count myself among the medical humanists, but I have no claim to counting myself yet among the practitioners of narrative medicine: this book is my first attempt.

The next twelve chapters will present what I recall from memory and from my notes of my interactions with twelve different, actual patients—not composites or hypotheticals—over the course of my 6 years with Pathways. I had generated an average of five notes per day, 100 days per year, for a total of 3000 on all my patients together, of which about a fifth informed the narratives that follow. I had filed them electronically on the day of each encounter. I began formulating the idea of this book during my last year of work there, and in anticipation of writing it, I brought these notes along on a flash-drive when I left.

I was fortunate during those years to be using one of the earlier versions of an electronic health record, which asked for documentation in the form of text, rather than of drop-down categories, and which therefore allowed me to capture conversations and observations of interest to me. More recent versions, which emphasize drop-down categories over text, are favored by emergency room physicians, accountants, and administrative reviewers, who, understandably, care more about objectives, goals, and services, which are required as of the first visit and useful for evaluating patients in emergency settings. But information in these categories changes little thereafter. I realize how fortunate I had been: such a version would not have been much help in this current effort.

I was to learn only on sitting down to begin to write, 4 years after my departure, just how impressionistic my memory was. I scrolled through it to select the patients to describe, but I was in for some surprises, when I consulted my notes. Sometimes these confirmed my recollections and were helpful anyway in providing the timeline of significant events and details of conversations. Regularly, they showed how long it took me to come up with a clear diagnosis and plan of action that satisfied both the patient and me, and my failures of understanding were not rare; indeed, I would probably have hesitated to be so forthcoming, earlier in my career, out of concern for my reputation. Even now I need to invoke the gracious acknowledgment by Kleinman (1988) of some of his mistakes and even of the verbal punishment he took for them, but I suspect more than a few other psychiatrists have also had similar experiences along the way. Sometimes, the notes even showed my impression to have been downright mistaken: to my disappointment I was forced to exclude the narrative I had written about one cordial and appreciative man, who did make some significant progress in his personal life, but who never managed to do so in relation to his repeatedly stated goals of work and of general health management.

I have tried to remain as faithful to the actual encounters and events as I could; thus, the only fictional element comes from my having tried to impose some order on what were, in fact, merely sequential, real-life encounters. I was a character in each of these narratives, and now I am the narrator for all of them. It seems to me that the professionals most identified with embedding themselves in cultures of work or healing and with providing accounts of them are the anthropologists. Among them I am indebted to Kleinman, the pioneer here, and to one of his protégés, Mattingly (1998). She cites Aristotle as having distinguished narrative from everyday life by the former's having given a plot to the events of the latter. Then she does him one better: she says people in general need narratives so badly that they use their own, both to direct their own actions in the first place and then to "find the story" in what they are observing. Later she goes on to assert that a "hopeful therapeutic plot" arises from the need which suffering patients have for "some hope for success, some reason to take a risk." And she wishes for healers the power to describe their work through narrative, "rather than the flattened prose of biomedical discourse." She ascribes that power, fairly enough, to Robert Coles and to the late Oliver Sacks. To those two I would add Sigmund Freud and D.W. Winnicott. Those four have set a very high bar, indeed.

It is of course impossible to discount my own cultural bias, since, as I have been taught, each of us sees the world, and thus distorts it, through the prism of her/his own culture. T.E. Lawrence, who may be considered one of the most qualified to write about the issue of trying to see the world through two different cultures, found that whenever he came close to doing so, "then madness was very near (Lawrence 1935)." But in my effort I am comforted by something Kleinman taught me and my fellow NYS-OMH psychiatrists in an interactive teleconference on cultural sensitivity that aired the late 1990s. He explained that, since each of us is culturally unique, once age and social class and gender are added into the mix along with ethnicity, teaching cultural sensitivity is futile. Instead, he suggested we try what he learned from his own clinical work, where he inquires, at intervals throughout an interview, whether he has got right what the patient is trying to tell him about the patient's various relationships and roles. One example he used was, "Is that what you mean about what your father expected of you?"

Of course, in presenting these narratives to you as examples of recovery, I am imposing plots that were not apparent at the beginning of my work with any patient. That is not only because I could not tell from the outset whether recovery would occur; it is also because the plots necessarily came from the patients themselves, not from me. I have tried to distinguish the events from their significance, which was often evident only later. You will see that I do not present the details of patients' developmental histories or prior mental health histories at the beginning of the narratives of patients who were already at Pathways when I arrived, because I reviewed these details only cursorily at the outset, and also because I was usually plunging into the middle of ongoing treatment, which I did not want to interrupt. Thus, these retrospective narratives will eventually reveal information that I acquired only over the course of treatment. Partly, this way of acquiring information reflected my faith that, when it emerged, it would do so in meaningful connections to current issues, so that its significance would stand out more clearly; but partly, it may have been a mistake, since, in my private practice, I always elicit such information in the first meeting, as a way of determining whether we are a suitable match and to set a course of treatment. Others of these narratives present patients who came to Pathways after I did and so began their treatment with me. With them I did start from the beginning, and so I present more of their initial information up-front. You can judge for yourself which you prefer. Either way, it seemed to me that the earlier experiences they described had meaning only in the context of ongoing interactions and events.

I should alert you here to something you may find missing from someone who was psychoanalytically trained, even if not certified, and that is, any attempts to interpret what my patients were trying to tell me. That is because I do not think that way when I am working; rather, I expect them to tell me whatever concerns them at the time and assume that they mean what they say. What is important to them at a deeper level will become clear over time, because they will return to those concerns again and again.

This is the same approach I try to teach students in general medicine in regard to psychiatric issues they may encounter in patients on general medical units: forget their psychiatric issues and concentrate on the general medical symptoms that brought them there in the first place, as would be appropriate for any patient without psychiatric issues (Section "My Personal Career Trajectory, Leading up to Outreach Psychiatry"). My own induction into this perspective was conveyed to me by a patient I was introduced to while rotating through an obstetrical unit during medical school. "Here's one for you!" announced the resident performing the delivery, knowing of my interest in psychiatry, while flashing her psychiatric chart at me, which was thicker than a telephone book. "Please just hold my hand," said the woman, and I did, while she proceeded to go through a series of rock-hard pelvic contractions without requiring any anesthesia. "Thank you" was all she said when it was over. The resident was impressed.

Another patient taught me what can happen if the physician takes the converse approach. A woman whom I was treating for a stable bipolar illness was scheduled to undergo a hysterectomy because of hemorrhaging uterine fibroids, and we discussed her expectations and concerns. Then the procedure was canceled at the last moment, because the gynecologic surgeon decided she would present behavioral problems during her recovery. My appeals to him and to my own department chairman were of no avail: the patient received radium implants instead of surgery. Two years later I attended her funeral: she had died of complications of abdominal adhesions, caused by the local radiation.

Each of the 12 narratives that follows has a simple arc: the patient was initially unstable, and nearly all had become homeless for a considerable period, after coming from prolonged or episodic hospitalization, sometimes along with incarceration; then the conflicts which maintained the instability were clarified and to some degree resolved; and finally, the patient settled into her/his new and preferred routine, which included managing the illness, as only one issue among many. The abstracts at the beginning of each narrative are intended to highlight both the generic issues applicable to many patients, and the specific issues reflective of the particular patient's life goals, conflicts, and personal assets.

My work was a clinical service, not a research enterprise, so I gathered no statistical data. Still, my impression is that the 12 narratives here represent the half or so of my patients whom I would judge as having made significant progress toward recovery. Many of the others did engage with the same issues but did not enjoy the same degree of success. I will try to bring you into the settings and into the events of their lives, so that you can judge my observations for yourselves, especially those about the nature of recovery. At the end of each of the narratives I will add a postscript, describing my best efforts at contacting them for their consent to publish my narrative of what they had accomplished during the period when we met, and containing what I learned of their experiences and status over the nearly 5 years since I had last seen them. Of the nine survivors I was able to learn directly or from family that eight were functioning as well or better than I would have predicted from our work together. In the last chapter, before drawing conclusions about outreach psychiatry, I will give an accounting of those patients whom I believe did not benefit particularly from my interactions with them or with our team, and who were, after as much as 6 years, pretty much at the same level of functioning as when we began. Feel free to second-guess me.

Confidentiality and Consent Issues

As stated above, I will present real individuals, not composites. I have chosen this approach because, when I read composites in the professional literature, they seem to illustrate general issues rather than actual lives, and verisimilitude is crucial to my goals here. None of my patients is a public figure; nevertheless, the portraits will be clearly recognizable to themselves, their respective families, their fellow-patients, and some Pathways staff from 2005–2011. Anonymity among this small group would be impossible.

Nearly 5 years after I left Pathways, my plan was to reconnect with each of them
—or in the case of the three who were deceased (all from potentially preventable
general medical causes), with a close relative—both to record their current status
and to obtain their consent to publish the narratives I had written. In this effort I was
materially assisted by administrators at two other agencies in New York City,
Services for the Underserved (SUS) and Post-Graduate Center for Mental Health
(PGCMH), who together had taken over the care and treatment of the former clients
of Pathways' Jamaica team at the beginning of 2015. These agencies have been
providing their own brand of supported housing and some outreach services since
long before Pathways was founded. They have their own perspectives on the factors
promoting or inhibiting recovery, and they will continue to play an important role in
developing them further.

Two of my former patients were receiving supported housing services from
PGCMH. One of them responded to my phone call and met with me several times.
The other had recently suffered from the emergence of severe new symptoms, so the
team leader requested I not contact him, pending further notice, although those may
yet turn out to remit. A third patient of mine, I was delighted to discover, was on the
staff at SUS. One relative of a deceased patient declined to return my several calls,
and I was unable to locate any close family member for a second; the relative of the
third provided consent after reviewing my narrative, which I had sent her by e-mail.
Through their telephone numbers, which I had kept in my notes, or from those I had
recorded for the psychiatrists or clinics I had referred them to upon their discharge
from Pathways, I was able to contact five of the remaining six of my patients, and a
close relative of the sixth. I was able to locate all nine who survived and a close
family member for two of the three who were deceased; however, not all of the
eleven chose to respond to my inquiries. Ultimately, six of my patients, along with
the relative of a seventh, who was deceased, provided consent. For the five I could
not contact, and for one who requested it, I changed their actual names, to protect
their privacy. This practice conforms, insofar as it was possible for me to do so, to
accepted practice in presenting such reports (Brettell 1993).

For better or for worse I resisted the temptation to recast any of the narratives in
the light of these updates.

References

Bleuler E (1911) Dementia Praecox oder Gruppe der Schizophrenien. Deuticke, Leipzig (English
    edition: Bleuler E (1950). Dementia Praecox or the Group of Schizophrenias (trans: Zinkin J)).
    International Universities Press, New York
Brettell CB (1993) When They Read What We Write: The Politics of Ethnography. Bergin &
    Garvey, Westport
Davidson L, Harding C, Spaniol L (eds) (2005) Recovery from Severe Mental Illnesses: Research
    Evidence and Implications for Practice, vol 1. Center for Psychiatric Rehabilitation, Boston
Eldred DM, Brooks GW, Deane WN, Taylor MB (1962) The rehabilitation of the hospitalized
    mentally ill—the Vermont story. Am J Public Health Nation's Health 52(1):39–46

Flannery M, Glickman M (1996) Fountain House: Portraits of Lives Retrieved from Mental Illness. Hazelden, Center City

Gladwell M (2006) Million Dollar Murray. New Yorker, Feb 2013

Harding CM, Brooks GW, Ashikaga T, Strauss JS, Breier A (1987) The Vermont longitudinal study of persons with severe mental illness I: methodology, study sample, and overall status 32 years later. Am J Psychiatry 144:718–726

Kane JM, Robinson DG, Schooler NR et al (2015) Comprehensive versus usual community care for first-episode psychosis: 2-Year outcomes from the outcomes outcomes NIMH RAISE early treatment program. Am J Psych 172:237–248

Kleinman A (1988) The Illness Narratives. Basic Books (Harper Collins), USA, p 139

Kraepelin E (1883) Compendium der Psychiatrie: Zum Gebrauche fuer Studierende und Aertze [Compendium of Psychiatry: For the Use of Students and Physicians]

Lawrence TE (1935) Seven Pillars of Wisdom. Doubleday, Garden City, p 32

Lifton R (1973) Home from the War. Simon and Schuster, New York

Mattingly C (1998) Healing Dramas and Clinical Plots: The Narrative Structure of Experience. Cambridge University Press, p 7

Searles H (1961) Phases of patient-therapist interaction in the psychotherapy of chronic schizophrenia. Brit J Med Psychol 34:169–193

Stein LI, Test MA (1980) Alternative to mental hospital treatment. I. Conceptual model, treatment program, and clinical evaluation. Arch Gen Psychiatry 37:392–397

Tsemberis S, Eisenberg RF (2000) Pathways to housing: supported housing for street-dwelling homeless individuals with psychiatric disabilities. Psychiatric Serv 51(4):487–493; see also: Padgett DK, Henwood B, Tsemberis S (2015) Housing First: Ending Homelessness, Transforming Systems, and Changing lives. Oxford University Press, New York

Tucker W (2007) How People Change: The Short Story as Case History. The Other Press, New York

Chapter 2
Gary N.

Personal and Psychiatric History

Gary N. had joined the Pathways roster only a few months before I began my tenure there, in March, 2005. He was fresh off the streets—or rather, the subways, the "F" line having been his favorite. I was to learn later, when he would report returning there during periods of stress, that he was fond of it, not only because it offered him warmth in winter and coolness in summer, but also because alcohol and drugs and, especially, smoking were prohibited there, so that he was effectively protected from his urges. Indeed, it was unclear why he had agreed to join our program at all: we were offering him his own apartment, but he had been given housing in the past, only to lose it, by throwing loud "crack" parties, and by letting undesirables in. He knew he remained at risk of repeating these behaviors. He had to endure occasional, brief hospitalizations when paranoid symptoms unmasked by substance abuse caught up with him, but these cleared quickly without deleterious consequences. He was vulnerable to arrest for turnstile jumping and public urination, and he could hardly afford the fines that he accrued for these infractions, but the police were not pursuing him or threatening him with prosecution or prison. Thus, what he was looking for was not immediately apparent, and it was only gradually, over the course of the 6 years we would spend getting to know each other, that I came to realize that he had his own, quite private agenda, which I will get to, shortly.

Furthermore, as you are about to learn, Gary had many accomplishments under his belt before becoming disabled, and many personal assets, such as politeness, sociability, warmth, and affection for women, with several of whom he had intimate relationships. His major disability, the one that knocked him off the satisfactory course his life had taken previously, was the emergence of his severe vulnerability to substance abuse and, when abusing, to irascibility, sometimes leading to fights. So, you may be wondering, why is his narrative the first in this series? If he did not cost the public systems very much, and if he had once managed on his own, would he not do so again, even without intensive outreach services? Yet, as you will see,

© Springer International Publishing Switzerland 2016
W. Tucker, *Narratives of Recovery from Serious Mental Illness*,
DOI 10.1007/978-3-319-33727-2_2

he was not heading in a positive direction at all; rather, like so many with chronic relapsing substance abuse, his life was heading downwards, as he was the first to recognize. In fact, he illustrates many of the issues around diagnosis, appropriate medication, treatment philosophy, and setting his own goals for treatment that are relevant to any unstable patient.

Gary was 49 when we met, 55 when I left Pathways. He was a wiry, light-skinned black man of average height and weight. For some time he dressed casually and unremarkably, but later on he would frequently show up in a suit and tie, as if to let me know he was doing better. He spoke in a casual, low-key manner, but his vocabulary indicated both intelligence and sophistication. He was invariably polite with me and modulated in his tone. Yet, it was not only his reports of responding with physical violence to being crossed or abused, but also something in his manner, that commanded respect. He exuded both sensitivity and quiet strength.

At our first meeting, he presented an array of common problems, such as dissatisfaction with a substance-abusing housemate, his own impulses to relapse, and financial straits, but at the end he came up with an unexpected one: a corn on one of his toes, which hurt when he walked. I decided to focus on this last one, hoping to accomplish something concrete that would get us off to a good start. So, I asked him to take off his shoes and socks. Not letting on whether he was puzzled, he complied. There was the corn, hard and rough to the touch, and red around the edges. Since I did not know much podiatry, I simply suggested he soak his foot in Epsom salts and consider picking up some looser-fitting shoes. He assented, and I thought we had put one problem behind us and even reached some understanding of how we would proceed, one step at a time. But he had his own sense of that process, and I had a lot to learn.

I never tried to get much of a history of his development up through adolescence, but he told me something later that seemed to provide an insight into much of it. He remarked, "When my mother told me not to expect a bed of roses, I told her I knew she was bringing me only the thorns." I took this remark to mean that he had learned from the beginning that he could not fully trust even the person closest to him, as he told me his mother considered herself to be. That did not mean he was incapable of trust altogether, but rather, that he would have to deal circumspectly with close relationships and to hedge his bets, if he were to escape being hurt.

Knowing this from the start of our work would have helped me later to understand how he went about setting up two important, sustaining networks. One of these was his relationships with women: he fathered his first child by a girl when they were both in their mid-teens, whom he thereafter considered his wife, and with whom he had another child almost 30 years later. In between these he also had four other children by different high-school classmates. Though he had no regular contact with these other women later, he did occasionally look them up, and he was fondest, among all his children, of the daughter of one of them.

The other network, in some ways quite similar to the first, was the one he established while at Pathways. Besides our monthly visits he met weekly with our director of family therapy, Lascelles Black, a distinguished clinician-teacher whose background and wisdom I always assumed gave him greater insight into Gary than I could hope to gain; also regularly with our peer-specialist and substance abuse counselor, Ricardo Moore, a black man of great depth and talent; and also, frequently, with his older brother, himself a certified Gestalt therapist, who, it might have appeared, would have had the most leverage of the four of us.

Lest you jump to the conclusion that Pathways was extremely well-endowed with resources, let me assure you that this elaborate support system was entirely of Gary's making: each of us probably imagined that Gary was closest to one of the other three. Now, if I am correct, this feeling we may have had attests to Gary's genuine efforts to obtain help and support from us in spite of his own difficulties with trust, rather than to manipulate us: a manipulative person would have made each of us feel we were the special one, more important to him than the others. As his story unfolds, you will see how tactfully he managed to make appropriate use of each of us, while finding his own way forward, and how grateful he was when he believed he had made progress.

Gary's mother had died of alcoholism and an older brother suffered from it, and there is no question that Gary suffered from it as well, probably from adolescence, as his multiple intimate relationships may reflect. Nevertheless, during that same time period he learned to play the drums and earned some money with get-up bands. He also worked, in his mid-20s, for the city's sanitation department, where his continual rhythm-and-blues singing, while on the job, earned him the epithet of Singing Sanitation Man. Not surprisingly, his drinking caused him soon to lose that relatively lucrative and potentially secure position. Also in those years, when the "crack" form of cocaine became available, he began abusing that, as well; nevertheless, his crack use must not have been apparent, because in his early 30s he managed to pass screening and serve a full tour of duty in the Navy on a ship in the Mediterranean, leading up to Operation Desert Storm in 1991.

It was shortly after that tour ended, that he was first admitted to a psychiatric hospital, because of the emergence, in the context of heavy drinking and crack use, of paranoid delusions and assaultive behavior, including one episode in which he severely beat a man, leaving himself with a frightening memory he never wanted to reenact. From this or perhaps from a subsequent episode of the same configuration, Gary emerged with two things: the label of paranoid schizophrenia and the commitment to monthly injections of antipsychotic medication, supplemented by daily oral antipsychotic medication and by a medication for their side effects.

Treatment Begins

At least a substantial proportion of my psychiatric peers would support me in taking issue with Gary's diagnosis, in the absence of chronic psychotic symptoms, and therefore, with his prescribed treatment. Among our rationales would be the obvious diagnosis of substance abuse, which was adequate to explain his periodic irascibility; his family history of substance abuse in the absence of other serious mental illnesses; the favorable personal history of significant intimate relationships;

and the relatively late emergence, for schizophrenia, of his psychotic symptoms—
and even then, only in the context of alcohol and drug use. Since these medications
are fraught with neurological and metabolic side effects, a cost/benefit view would
suggest they not be prescribed over time unless clearly indicated.

Nevertheless, in accordance with an old principle that it is better to make major
changes only slowly, I waited until considerably later before bringing up the option
of reconsidering his diagnosis and medications. Somewhat to my surprise, he
explained that he considered his medications a reliable protection against relapse to
paranoid symptoms, and that he feared relapse to alcohol was such a likely even-
tuality that he wanted as much protection from the symptoms that might follow
from it as he could get. He reinforced his preference by adding that any shaking he
exhibited was due to drinking too much coffee and not to the medication. Somewhat
reluctantly, I went along with his request, reminding myself that no one who fails to
benefit from this type of medication asks for more of it.

Still, I continued to doubt his diagnosis of a psychotic illness. Eventually,
considering the episodic nature of his symptomatic episodes, I proposed to him that
he might be suffering from bipolar illness, which is itself frequently accompanied
by substance abuse. Tactfully, he replied that he did not mind a reconsideration of
his diagnosis. However, anticipating my suggestion that he try taking lithium, a
mood-stabilizer, instead of his antipsychotic medication, he assured me that he was
managing his money well, which was an explicit denial of the manic tendency to
overspend; moreover, he added that a friend had developed a dry mouth from taking
lithium, so he would rather not undergo a trial of it. I thought he was trying to tell
me that the specific diagnosis was not the point, and that I should just pick one that
would let me continue providing medication he needed. If so, he was addressing my
doubts quite effectively.

It was only when I finally began to see his symptoms from his point of view that
I came up with an acceptable improvement to his medication regimen. I was
puzzled by his reports of frequently forgetting to take one or the other of his two
oral medications, because he was so insistent on receiving them. Somehow, forgetting the medication for side effects resulted either in a bad night's sleep or the
disappointment of having let himself down. Confronting him would have made no
sense, so instead, I switched course and suggested we increase his monthly dose of
the injectable antipsychotic medication and discontinue the oral one. He was
delighted. Four months later he reported, "I don't antagonize people now; I'm
quiet." In subsequent months he added that he felt more comfortable and secure,
thus showing me that he had probably been correct in the first place about the need
for antipsychotic medication, perhaps to reduce his irritability. Even with his oral
medication for neurological side effects reduced to one pill, twice a day, he continued occasionally to forget it, each time still with regret. I believe that his struggle
to take medication regularly meant to him that he was doing something to tip the
balance in favor of his health.

Early on, he set the topics for our discourse: his continual temptation to relapse,
often stimulated by multiple offers from abusers seeking to lure him back to alcohol
and drugs; his efforts to save money on food, so that he could afford to purchase

coffee and cigarettes as replacements for substances of abuse; his intermittent efforts to reduce his smoking; and his need to restrict his coffee intake to the morning and afternoon hours, so that it would not interfere with his sleep. Surely, these were relevant to a person suffering primarily from substance abuse. But in addition I kept listening for his definition of progress toward personal goals. He tried to make our interactions comfortable for me by focusing on topics he knew from experience that psychiatrists preferred, namely, his symptoms, while he continued to struggle with his own impulsivity, not knowing himself for sure when the time to move on was at hand. Both of us continued trying to figure out the best pace, tactics, and strategies together.

In Gary's case you might think goal-setting would be obvious: if his problem was substance abuse, then quitting the abuse and maintaining abstinence must be his goal. Certainly, he had observed enough, from the demise of family members and fellow–patients, and from the chaos in the lives of those still abusing, including his own repeated job losses, to convince himself of what the alternative would bring. He had even been told by a physician, sometime along the way, that he had a "damaged liver" and was developing a "wet brain." But on his own he had largely given up abusing substances, even before coming to Pathways.

What remained, aside from occasional, brief relapses to alcohol, were the nagging temptations to return to his former life of continuous abuse. Why else would he have continued to focus on these temptations and his urges to resist them, reporting them at nearly half of our eventual total of 75 meetings? For example, he described the can of Budweiser placed before him by a fellow-resident of the YMCA as "clean, well-opened," a term good enough to pass for advertising copy, and one that conjured up the mouth-watering quality of the invitation. It would have been simpler to avoid the tempters altogether. He surely knew this, thanks to having intermittently attended meetings of Alcoholics Anonymous and Narcotics Anonymous, where he would have heard plenty about strategies to avoid the ubiquitous lure of drugs and dealers—what he called "being surrounded by Indians."

One easy answer would be that he had not yet decided that he was ready to give up substances of abuse, because his recent pattern had at least offered some structure and easy satisfactions, even if it was risky. Another would be that he was just stringing along the four of us most immediately involved with his care. A third would be that he did not yet have a clear idea of an alternative, after having spent at least half his life going downhill with only intermittent accomplishments, such as playing music and spending affectionate moments with women friends. But none of those would be my answer. I think he was not simply nostalgic for the good moments of his past, but also for the man he had been at his best, as a young adult, and wanted a second go-round to make a whole life out of more of those moments, better than he had, the first time. This, I believe, was his private agenda.

Even if he was exaggerating his musical achievements by claiming to have played back-up for James Brown and Michael Jackson, or to have family connections to Cab Calloway, Duke Ellington, or Charles Rangel, that would have been no worse than wishful thinking on his part. I believe he sized up the four of us

—Lascelles, Ricardo, his older brother, and me—well enough to understand our motivations and to match them against his own, borrowing what he could from each of us and putting it to use. Furthermore, he was continually searching for sources of information beyond us, explaining, for example, "I watch TV talk shows to learn how to talk better to people."

Course of Treatment

Now that you are acquainted with his personal style and methods, it is time to lay out what I considered his trajectory over the 6 years of our working together, so that you can judge his progress for yourself. Beyond the usual metrics for assessing it—symptom management, quality of personal relationships, self-care, and grooming, use of social supports—the one that seemed to subsume all these was his ability to make the most of each of his progressively more independent living situations. During the first 18 months of our meetings he lived with other patients in a house owned by Pathways; during the next 36 months he lived in the local YMCA; and during the last 18 months he lived in another house, with very different house-mates from the first time and with a very different outcome, much more successful than his first experience with housemates.

The initial rationale for assigning him to a house rather than to his own apart-ment was his claim that loneliness was a trigger for relapse to drugs and alcohol; however, throwing him together with a severe poly-substance abuser who flaunted his behavior and was also threatening, had put considerable stress on Gary's self-control. To combat these feelings, and to improve his spotty attendance at AA and NA meetings, he tried to join two other support organizations, Venture House, for help with substance abuse, and Transitional Services, Inc. (TSI), which provided not only employment support but also structured weekend programs, which Pathways, though on-call for emergencies, did not provide. But he could not meet the sustained sobriety requirement of the first, nor the requirement of the second for undergoing a thorough physical examination with follow-up laboratory tests, even after months of scheduled and broken appointments.

I did not consider his difficulty in meeting these requirements a sign of ambivalence, because he was so persistent in his attempts, but rather, of the struggle he was encountering in his effort to change the direction of his life. Those of us without the experience of addiction have trouble imagining how completely it takes over, and we appreciate retrospective accounts of success, where some factor or other is credited with bringing it about. But Gary enjoyed no such clear epiphany; rather, he languished until nearly the end of the 6 years in the transition back to a life without addiction, searching for another activity that would structure his life.

His efforts at self-care were similarly disappointing: his dentist told him he needed to undergo extraction of a rotten molar and of impacted wisdom teeth, but he bolted repeatedly from the dentist's office, even after receiving lidocaine anal-gesia, out of fear of the impending pain. No amount of advice or intervention by a qualified podiatrist could break the cycle of repeated bouts of foot pain. He continued to have trouble with impulsivity. Once, having forgotten his key, he put his hand through a window alongside the door of his house and sustained a thumb full of glass splinters. His clothing was often spotted, and he reported failing to brush his teeth. He dropped and broke the CD player his brother had gotten him, though listening to music was a rare source of diversion and pleasure. He sometimes bought beer with the food money his brother occasionally provided to him. He referred to all this behavior, philosophically, as his "homeless ways," but more ominously, he feared at times that he was actually "falling apart."

Improvement Begins

I do not recall who it was among the various team members and array of his supportive therapists who figured out that something had to be done. We occasionally referred patients to the local YMCA who needed more structure than what the standard, market-rate housing in the community provided. I knew it from visiting several of my patients whom we housed there temporarily, and Gary had visited several acquaintances there. Perhaps, he was the one who encouraged the idea. It was not an obvious choice for him, because there was an extensive list of house rules designating proscribed behaviors, in contrast to Pathways, where nearly any behavior that was not immediately dangerous was tolerated, in accordance with our policy of "harm reduction" (Section "The Pathways Model"). One of these rules specified that in-house drinking or illicit substance use would result in immediate expulsion.

In retrospect, I think Gary somehow realized even before he moved in that structure—rules and physical barriers—to help him avoid being provoked, was precisely what he needed. He thrived on it, working with or around each rule so adroitly that he was never, over the course of his three-year stay at the YMCA, threatened with expulsion. This was a measure of success I am not sure that anyone on our team would have bet on his achieving at the time of his moving in. He drank beer occasionally, but never on the premises and never to excess. He had no opportunity to let in undesirables, because security personnel screened every visitor. He rejected successive offers of drugs, accompanied by appealing displays of drug paraphernalia, more easily than he could have in the street, because he could always retreat to his room without fear of reprisal. Moreover, through politeness and persistence he managed to cadge leftover food from the dining room staff, so that he did not have to spend all his meager monthly allotment to sustain himself and, thereby, had some disposable income in reserve, so as to preserve some necessary autonomy in the context of giving up his habitual indulgences.

All these changes may appear to you to be only slight modifications of the behaviors he exhibited previously, but to him they represented a distancing from his former habits and a space in which to try out new and more sustainable ways of engaging with his social environment, both inside and outside the YMCA. He succeeded in undergoing the necessary tooth extractions and was pleased to have required no more analgesia than aspirin for the post-operative pain. He began attending TSI programs regularly on weekends, "to keep out of trouble," though he never managed to achieve full membership status. He showed up in criminal court to be arraigned on his misdemeanor charges and to settle them. He learned, thanks to his brother, to shop in supermarkets rather than in corner groceries, in order to obtain food that was not only fresher and more varied but also less expensive. He tried working in maintenance for Pathways and, though he shortly gave it up, saying that he did not yet feel ready to return to work, he added that his disability status "isn't forever." He reported multiple meetings with some of his former girlfriends and expressed pleasure in talking with them and occasionally receiving a kiss. Altogether, he reported one day, "I'm functioning like a human being in the community, for the first time since I was a kid, as if the sun had penetrated a stone wall."

During this period also, he began to feel freer about expressing what he thought of the communications between us. Like many patients he thought he was obligated to report either on progress he was making or on his regret for failing to do so. But now he felt comfortable expressing thoughts and feelings of his own choosing. "No one has a good day every day—not even you!" he put it once. Another time, he referred back to having told me about problems in his family of origin, such as another older brother's alcoholism, explaining, "I was trying to be real yesterday, talking about more than pills and appointments, to let out more than the candy-coated stuff, like my [short-lived] job."

While trying out this more open way of talking about his concerns, he began dressing more spiffily, sometimes in a suit and tie. He was experimenting with revealing more of himself through his appearance, his clothes sometimes being casual, sometimes formal; each outfit sometimes clean, sometimes spotted. He had reported that his brother had earlier accused him of letting himself go, and now, sometime later, Gary was responding by trying to take better care of himself, but the ongoing conflict over doing so was written all over him, as he dressed sometimes the old way, sometimes the new. Around the time he was moving out of the YMCA, some of his self-doubts caused him to avoid meeting with me for 2 months, in order to give himself time and space to figure out how much he wanted to reveal.

Smoking-cessation, as you may imagine, had emerged as a major goal, for the usual reasons of both cost and health. It took a considerable period of time to run through the various substitute routes for nicotine—gum, pills, patches—and various support groups, but this process did not achieve its aim, nor did it help with his secondary goal of structuring his time, as the pursuit of drugs had done. His principal success here was in restricting himself to picking up only cigarette butts from the sidewalk to smoke, rather than in purchasing "loosies [i.e., hand-rolled cigarettes, formed from loose tobacco]."

Each day was a struggle. Going in search of a cup of coffee may seem like a harmless enough activity, but he drank up to ten cups a day, enough to cause frequent nighttime urination, itself leading to a disturbing medical complication, which I will get to, shortly. Then his efforts switched to trying to reduce his coffee consumption, especially in the evenings. Attending harm-reduction group, waiting in line at the Medicaid office to renew his eligibility, following through on medical tests for his TSI application, and in-between, spending long hours in front of the TV—these were his ways of passing the time and staying out of trouble, but they hardly constituted a full life, and not having one was always dangerous for him.

To visit him in his room at the YMCA I had to sign in with security each time, take an elevator, and then wind my way down and around a series of hallways to reach his door. He was invariably welcoming. The room itself was not much wider than his single-bed cot, placed along a wall. The four walls were unadorned, but there was a window, fortunately, which he kept open, summer and winter, to let in fresh air and to let out some of the cigarette smell that permeated everything. Ashtrays, filled to overflowing, took up a good deal of the area of the only flat surface at his disposal: the top of a small refrigerator. Between the ashtrays lay opened, half-empty cans of tuna and jars of jam. There was a small microwave for warming pizza or coffee. Crushed soda cans were scattered about the floor, among cast-off shoes and socks, those unyielding causes of his tormented feet. He never failed to offer me a seat on his one chair, sitting down himself on the cot. After our talk he sometimes accompanied me to the elevator and down to the front door. I recall his having introduced me to a fellow-resident he dubbed Baryshnikov, because of his dancing ability, and pointed out the dining room on a lower floor, where he would show up after regular mealtimes to pick up leftovers. However modest they were, his living arrangements served their purpose.

It was hard for me to understand why he was invariably cheerful during these visits, when his grim surroundings saddened me. In retrospect, I suppose it was that all his energy went into resisting his addictive impulses, and he believed with justification that he was succeeding.

Six months into his three-year stay, he began to bring up the prospect of moving out. There was a distinct benefit to the rules and structure, he announced, but he would someday like an apartment of his own. The only problem was to decide when the right moment had arrived. He conceded that it would be hard for the Pathways staff, or even for him, to know that he was ready. Three months later, he brought up the prospect again, in the aftermath of having turned down the most recent offer of "appetizing" drugs, but he was aware that there was a larger problem, namely, how to fill his time in ways other than searching out or refusing offers of drugs and alcohol. Giving up knocking on doors to ask for handouts of coffee and cigarettes only freed up more time that he was uncertain how to fill. His feeling that he was doing better, that he was "not walking in the fog anymore," as he put it, alternated with doubts about his readiness.

As you will have come to expect from this narrative so far, Gary's proclivity for putting pressure on himself, even without involving substances of abuse, was considerable. Though his needs were modest to begin with, he managed to tempt fate, nearly 2 years into his stay, by borrowing small sums from local loan-sharks, something he referred to as having "gotten into a bit of mischief." Over 3 months he managed to run up sufficient small debts that he feared he would need to leave the YMCA precipitously to avoid being harmed in reprisal. Once again, his brother came through for him, paying off one debt in cash and replacing the CD player Gary had dropped and broken, so that he could use it to pay off the second and final one. "Now I don't have to take a trip" was how he summed it up.

Whether the episode with the loan-sharks was a warning that it was time to move out, or whether the relief and exhilaration over putting it behind him simply propelled him forward, he had convinced himself that the time had come. Several members of our treatment team had their doubts, as you may imagine, but we were all impressed with his continued avoidance of street drugs and with the overall success he had made of his tenure at the YMCA. Furthermore, it is our agency's policy to support our clients' efforts to move toward greater independence and responsibility, so we were inclined not to get in his way. Like him we were curious to see what would happen and were prepared to deal with the consequences. Our principal suggestion was that he consider moving into a house with three other Pathways clients, rather than to an apartment on his own, so that he would be less likely to experience the loneliness that had triggered relapse in the now-receding past. He accepted this suggestion willingly.

Gary's move from the YMCA into a house Pathways owned in the local community opened the curtain on the last phase of our work together. I knew that my time was gradually running out, because I had planned to retire from this strenuous work when I turned 70, just 2 years down the road. I had told my employer and a few fellow team members of my intention, but none of them gave much credence to an event announced so far in advance, and for our clients, so much is uncertain anyway from day-to-day, that time pressure is the least of their worries. Nor was there any desire on our part to put pressure on Gary to make good on his claim that he was ready to take on more responsibility for the course of his life: it was simply up to him to see what he could do. In retrospect, though, it appeared that he had given himself precisely that sort of challenge.

There was no way either of us could have anticipated that major losses to his support network were also about to occur, outside our respective abilities to prevent them. In fairly short order he lost, first, Lascelles Black as his primary therapist, an indirect casualty of the state funding shortfall from the recession of 2007–9; second, his substance abuse counselor, peer-specialist Ricardo Moore, who died tragically of cancer, just after passing his examination to become a Certified Alcoholism and Substance Abuse Counselor; and third, some degree of the regular support he received from his brother, whether out of personal reasons or of his sense that it was time to let Gary stand on his own.

Shortly after Gary's arrival at the house, an event occurred which served as a propitious warning for him. One of the three housemates living there at the time, who suffered from the most devastating and unremitting case of alcoholism I have ever encountered, died from it. Gary was shaken, but at least, neither of his two remaining housemates had any problems with substance abuse, nor would Pathways consider placing any such person with him in the future. The desire for peaceful co-existence with those two housemates put a gentle brake on his self-destructive impulses not dissimilar to the firm one imposed by the house rules at the YMCA.

Consolidation of Gains; New Capacities

In a development that had farther-reaching benefits both for Gary and for me than I could have anticipated at the time, I took up a position where I had more regular contact with him and more access to information on how he was managing. Besides being the psychiatrist for all three remaining housemates individually, I became party to their interactions when they eagerly accepted my offer to serve as coordinator of their monthly house meetings, knowing better than I that issues would quickly arise. Following, these meetings Gary regularly asked if he could drive back to the Pathways office with me. In the van he would talk about his familiarity with the neighborhood where his current house was located, not far from where he had grown up, and about his on-again-off-again relationship with an elderly aunt, for whom he sometimes performed chores in return for a meal, but who laid down strict rules of behavior as a condition of these invitations.

Once I accompanied him and a few fellow-patients to a Mets baseball game. Third-base grandstand seats were still only $10! On the way home he reported having enjoyed it, but he had found it difficult to avoid having a beer, as he saw so many other fans doing; instead, he smoked steadily, to curb his alcohol craving. From such a vantage point it became clear to me quickly that changes were occurring. The past themes were to play out once again, but with significantly more favorable outcomes.

The house itself was indistinguishable, on the outside, from other one-family houses on the quiet residential block, but inside, it was not as well maintained as they probably were. The front door buzzer was nonfunctional, so that it was necessary to bang on the door to announce one's arrival. The individual bedrooms, arranged around a stairwell on the second floor, were small and under-furnished, so each man had to make piles of his belongings along the walls. The one bathroom was regularly cleaned by a Pathways employee, and there were no personal items visible on the sink or in the cabinet. There was almost no food on the kitchen shelves, so they looked bare and a bit too clean for comfort. It was the sparseness and quiet that characterized the common rooms, as well. The living room furniture was spare. A leatherette couch and a few wooden chairs, one of them, for some reason, a rocker, were scattered about, so that, for our monthly meetings, one of the men had to pull up all the chairs that were available to the one, small, all-purpose wooden table. The men did not often use the room to converse or spend time together, but rather, to listen to music, one at a time.

Despite these limitations there is no question that for Gary it was a step up. His room was certainly more spacious than the previous one at the YMCA, and he maintained it more neatly, free of food items, and spacious enough for his somewhat wider selection of clothing. Besides serving as a retreat, this one was also a point of pride. Other improvements were on their way.

This time around, his struggle against the temptation to resume drinking took on significance for his two housemates. On multiple occasions, Gary invited in, as a drinking companion, an acquaintance of his who was both dangerous and unpredictable, the perfect avatar of what he had been, himself, at his worst, and the foil for who he was becoming. The topic at our monthly house meetings moved from whether to let any strangers enter, to who was responsible in the moment for keeping strangers out by locking the door, and finally, to the need to get the lock itself fixed. Discussion of these very real, concrete topics took several months, during which Gary came around to share the view of his two housemates, namely, that all three of them were afraid of this particular, knife-wielding stranger, and therefore, that he should not be let in at all, nor allowed to sneak in through a front door left unlocked through negligence. Pathways obliged us by sending in a locksmith, and that settled the matter. This became the framework for settling subsequent issues.

The next hot topic was how to settle differences over private property. Seth, whom you will meet later (Chap. 9) accused Gary of stealing his MetroCard, to which Gary, to my surprise, openly acknowledged his guilt, justifying his action by accusing Seth of helping himself to Gary's food from the common refrigerator. In his view taking the card was more of an "exchange" than a theft. Here, the issue did not revolve around locks: each man had his own room, and there were common living areas, but in-house security could only be insured by common agreement. Trust, an unreliable element in most situations of life, did not enter into the calculation, because each man knew what was his and could easily enough make a tally. Once again, after discussions identified each of these concerns, there was agreement, and, to everyone's relief, it proved enduring, just as it continued to do over the issue of intruders.

With the next topic you will notice a diminishing trend from threats down to mere sources of friction. Gary stood accused of playing his radio loudly in the morning, thus disturbing the sleep of the others. Once again, he acknowledged his behavior, this time countercharging that their third housemate occasionally still left the front door unlocked. He added that, if that housemate made more of an effort, he would not mind preserving the morning quiet, because he, too, preferred to sleep later.

Now, if you have ever been a party to conflict resolution, including as a mediator, you know that when it succeeds, it is a heady tonic to all parties. But it is even more satisfying, when one of the parties has a history, much to his own chagrin, of having reacted violently to past provocations. Manifestations of actual camaraderie followed. When Gary's brother gave him a turkey to cook up for Thanksgiving, he invited his housemates to partake. This was a pleasant surprise to me, since Gary had informed me in no uncertain terms that any gifts from his brother were for him alone. When their third housemate repeatedly plugged up the kitchen sink, out of inattention, Gary made no fuss over repeatedly unplugging it. It sounded almost affectionate when he recounted, describing their third house-mate, "We haven't had any more complaints from our neighbor about his spraying the garden hose on her house." These deceptively routine events took on meaning because of the low level of personal interaction otherwise. As he put it, in his own special fashion, "We're on the other side of the clock now."

I would like to think of his use of the first-person plural as a reference to himself among those in recovery. The proscription against associating with people connected with one's abusing world is well known, but how, in fact, is someone in recovery to replace them? I think Gary was considering the need to do this, all along, and by making these compromises with his housemates, he was making the necessary leap.

I believe that in the context of these changes in his expanded living arrangements and diminished therapeutic supports, Gary was also figuring out new ways to use me. For example, a new physical problem arose that was reminiscent of our first exchanges around his corns, but potentially much more serious. Unable to curb his late-evening coffee consumption, and disturbed by having to make frequent nighttime trips to the bathroom as a consequence, he had consulted a private local physician. Why he had not gone back to his primary care physician at the neighborhood Medicaid clinic, who knew him better, I never inquired; perhaps, it was just a matter of a shorter waiting time. The private physician had given him a prescription for a medication to reduce urinary frequency, and over the ensuing month, Gary noticed a disturbing, swelling of both legs. He was considering consulting another private physician.

I knew he had some chronic asthma and congestion, as a result of his smoking, for which the Medicaid physician treated him intermittently; however, I had not heard anything about heart failure, the usual cause of leg edema. So, with the coincidence of the new medication and the new symptom, I suggested that he first simply try discontinuing the medication, to see whether the swelling would subside, before returning to the prescriber or looking elsewhere. To our mutual relief, the swelling disappeared, as quickly as it had come on. This outcome was for him as dramatic as the outcome for my consultation on my patient with pica early on in my tenure with NYS-OMH (Section "My Personal Career Trajectory, Leading up to Outreach Psychiatry"). A month later, Gary acknowledged that he was impressed by my diagnosis and intervention, which spared him considerable worry. The bottom line on the successful outcome of this incident, I believe, was that this was a problem that he himself believed needed a solution, in contrast to the one involving his corns, which I had seized upon for my own purposes, and which he could manage well enough on his own.

Even as we were now in the middle of our sixth year of working together, I could not be sure of what Gary thought of me, or, more to the point, what he considered to be my value to him. In my private practice it is fairly easy to answer this question, because the patients can discontinue their visits, whether they are paying directly or through a third party. But in a health-provider agency like Pathways, where I was the only psychiatrist for the team, patients had no such choice. Thus, it was from Gary's references to his other therapists, who were truly gifted, and for whom I had great personal and professional respect, that I was left to infer how he regarded us, perhaps, collectively.

Though he had not responded spontaneously to Ricardo Moore's death when it occurred, he now, in retrospect, brought up how helpful Ricardo had been to him around his substance abuse problems. It was not so much a matter of whether this assessment was true in practical terms, because Gary had discontinued crack on his own before ever coming to Pathways, and on the other hand alcohol never remained far from his mind. Rather, it was Ricardo's value as a role model that counted: here was a man who had pulled his own life together and had forged a viable future for himself.

Regarding his feelings for Lascelles Black, he drove the point home. His first reference was in the form of a denial: no, it was not due to Lascelles' departure that he had engaged in some drinking with their persistent intruder, the previous evening. The next time, it was more direct: would I consent to hold our regular meetings at a particular site near the Pathways office, where he and Lascelles used to meet? You will recall his difficulties with issues of trust, in contrast to which, this request stands out as an exception. One day, near the end of our time together, as we drove along in the van to his preferred meeting-place, he was able to report with genuine pleasure and delight that he had heard from another team-member that Lascelles had been asking how he was getting along. Such were the feelings Gary had sought to engender in those he cared for but whom he felt he had so often disappointed in the past.

To answer the question of whether these 6 years represent progress in Gary's life, it is first necessary to formulate your idea of who he was, by personality and assets, and therefore, of who he could still become, even in his 50s, if he could overcome a significant disability. As an initial approach, you might consider what it would take for him to continue to pursue sobriety, particularly in light of his habit of treading dangerously close to the line of falling back. He gave some hints, as when he said he was not ready to take on the responsibility of regularly being available to figure in the lives of any of his children, or to jettison his disability status; however, in mentioning them he showed that those steps had at least crossed his mind. He had been away from playing music too long to look forward to returning to it as a career, but playing with old acquaintances again would not be an unreasonable expectation. How gratifying was his brother's, or his own wife's, or his daughter's esteem, and would that motivation suffice? It was possible that the serious health risk posed by his heavy smoking might foreshorten his future, before he could pursue any of these other commitments.

But in the meantime he had learned how to make compromises and avoid taking offense, so as to be able to pursue at least limited social relationships in the context of a quieter but more sustainable life, meeting occasionally with women he had long known and some members of his family, and thinking back and forward to music and possibly to work. I think he had found himself again, and doing so was his goal from the beginning.

Post-script

At the time of trying to contact Gary to request his consent I learned from Lascelles Black that he had died of lung cancer about 2 years earlier, while still a Pathways client. I obtained the telephone number of his older brother, the licensed therapist mentioned in the narrative, and left messages on his voicemail multiple times; however, he chose not to return my calls. I asked Lascelles, who had met with Gary's brother several times, to intercede, and I believe he did so, but I still received no call from the brother. In the absence either of consent or of any refusal of it, I changed the first name and initial to protect his anonymity.

Chapter 3
Pamela P.

You may recall that my view of the primary role of the outreach psychiatrist is to hold onto the patient's coattails without any preconceived agenda, long enough for the patient to begin to use her/him as an aid to moving back onto, or finding the way onto, the path to personal goals (Section "My View of How These Patients Change"). This second narrative, illustrating the route that Pamela took to find her way onto a new, calmer, and sustainable work and life path, aims to illustrate just how much persistence that role demands, and at the same time, how rewarding that persistence can be, not only for the psychiatrist but also for the patient. The unexpected focus which this route followed for her was the emergence of an initially subtle, then explosive and prolonged, but finally resolved, general medical condition, hyperthyroidism.

Personal and Psychiatric History

When I first met her, Pamela was a single, black woman in her early 40s, who had already been living in a two-bedroom apartment provided by Pathways for three years. Four years previously, she had become homeless for a time and was ultimately directed to mental health care by a family court judge, in the course of addressing some issues between her and her daughter's father. The judge recommended strongly that she take an antipsychotic medication, and she had duly complied, taking olanzapine ever since.

She explained at our first meeting that she wanted to return to part-time work as an office assistant/store-cleaner, which the team's employment specialist was helping her to do. She requested that I reduce her medication dosage, because it caused her both considerable weight gain and, she claimed, an intermittent hand tremor, though the latter was not apparent. Her other medications included Benadryl, an antihistamine, which she needed to induce sleep, and quarterly injections of a birth control preparation she believed protected her from further

© Springer International Publishing Switzerland 2016
W. Tucker, *Narratives of Recovery from Serious Mental Illness*,
DOI 10.1007/978-3-319-33727-2_3

disappointment of the kind that her two children were causing her. She described how she tried to keep in touch with her 12-year-old daughter, who lived with her father in Las Vegas, by sending gifts, though in fact, despite both our efforts over the six years we were to work together, there was to be only one reply from the daughter. This estrangement was to persist as a source of great sadness to her, ultimately to be manifested, graphically, on her body.

To say that her appearance was striking would be an understatement. Though her clothing was modest and unremarkable, her bodily decorations were another story. She consistently chose wigs in bright colors—orange or yellow or green, fashioned of thick cloth strands without any pretense of looking natural. Her nails sometimes extended up to four inches in length and were invariably neatly and colorfully painted. These consistent features were accompanied by an array of numerous facial piercings, many with silver rings through lips, nose, and eyelids, but these varied in number, as if shifting with her moods. Only in conversation would you pick up on the fourth and most characteristic feature of all, namely, her invariable reference to herself in the second person, for example, "You [meaning she, herself] need to have a cavity filled next week."

All these idiosyncratic features belied her consistent effort, as she put it, "to lead a quiet life," which, in fact, she did, even though she acknowledged some wilder escapades earlier on, including trials of street drugs and, perhaps, of promiscuity. Her determination to leave those earlier ways behind was reflected in her statements that, "You've got to be careful that they put a ring on your finger [i.e., before having sex]," which reflected her earlier experience of being taken advantage of and helped explain her adherence to long-acting birth control medication.

It was not difficult to understand, in view of this history and, perhaps, of the judge's impression, why the Pathways team considered her to have a chronic psychosis, and even why, at a later point, when her behavior appeared to become more erratic, they attributed it to drug-taking. However, from our earliest months together onwards, I never saw any sign either of the first or of the second of these diagnoses. Though her appearance and manner of speaking were certainly unique and striking, her behavior, insofar as her interactions with me or other team members went, was consistent and intelligible; even more important, her thinking was invariably clearly organized and goal-directed, even when, as was to happen, her motivations took some empathic interpreting to understand. To check this view, I periodically consulted our art therapist, Rachel Romero, who was always pleased to volunteer samplings of Pamela's drawings from their weekly group meetings, highlighting not only their merit but also their excellent organization, thereby providing some confirmation of my own impression.

Pamela's striking appearance and unusual personality style showed in brilliant color how she felt about herself and how she wanted others to understand her. If you want to assume that these must have reflected some serious internal disorganization, go ahead, but you will never get to know her, and you will thereby be missing out on a lot. I only came to doubt my initial diagnosis of her once, as you shall soon learn, and that turned out to be due to a failure of imagination on my part. Nevertheless, you will have to judge from your own experience whether I was over-identifying with her in underestimating her psychopathology, or whether some of my team members were jumping reflexively to unsupported conclusions that overestimated it.

Treatment Begins

In contrast to Gary's (Chap. 2) the goal-setting process with her was straight forward—that is, until an unanticipated and threatening problem emerged. It focused on several practical, measurable issues. She was concerned about having gained over 30 lb on olanzapine, about wanting a smaller apartment that would justify her dismissing her current roommate, about not working, and, above all, as noted above, about reestablishing communication with her then 12-year-old daughter.

Within our first year, we had made some adjustments that seemed, gradually, to be clarifying her situation. Based on some comfort with her stability, on and off olanzapine, in varying doses, I was increasingly confident that she did not have either a chronic or a relapsing psychosis. The symptom she endorsed was anxiety, the origin of which was still not clear to either of us. For this there were many alternatives to olanzapine, and there was little risk in trying some of them. Her mannerisms and flamboyant appearance, it seemed, were probably attributable to a heightened personality style characterized by a tendency to display a lot of idiosyncratic thinking, speech, and behavior. The practical consequence of this diagnosis, which does not imply any lapses into disorganized thinking or psychosis, was that the value of medication to address it was pretty much up to her. She continued to want to take her usual medication and was pleased that the reduction in dose seemed to be working. She proceeded, stepwise, to lose nearly 100 lb, from her high of 235 down to her usual weight of around 140. Because she continued to report feeling well and pleased with the weight loss, I attributed it to my having reduced her medication, and I did not pay sufficient attention to what else might have caused it and how pronounced it was becoming. That oversight could have proven costly, but, as so often happens in medical practice, it did not: we both lucked out.

The issue of what to do with her tenant/roommate of about three years, who may also have been her boyfriend for a time, took us a while to untangle, but in the end resolved itself without complications. As long as he resided with her, he served as a source of information when he became concerned about her behavior. Because he was generally discreet and supportive, she mostly tolerated his presence.

Arrangements like this are by no means uncommon, and any "housing first" program needs to confront the issue of whether to make rules interdicting them. They are usually entered into by our clients in order to acquire some supplementary income. Pathways' concern focused—appropriately, in my opinion—on whether the arrangement was harmful to our client (Chap. 6) or disturbing to the client's neighbors (Section "Risks of Physical Harm to Outreach Clinicians"). As neither of these issues presented itself here, we did not interfere. Even so, she was comforted, as were other clients of ours, by having us for backup in the event that they might want to terminate such arrangements. Pamela reflected that, in the near future, she might call on us to do just that, if he did not vacate the apartment when she was ready for him to do so. This event was not to occur for another year, during which there was much back-and-forth deliberation on her part, because he acceded to her requests to increase his monthly payment, whenever she requested them.

She had pointed out his room to me on one of my visits to her apartment, but I had had no direct contact with him, until, about a year into my work with her, he called to inform me that she was behaving strangely, speaking gibberish, and had called the police to report what seemed to him to have been a hallucination. Since this call came on the heels of my team's view that she was using crack, the pressure was definitely on me to make an assessment. My first response was to confront her with the team's suspicion, and thereupon, she had no trouble expressing herself clearly, without so much as becoming agitated. She asserted, "No, you're (i.e., "I'm") not bizarre. The only crack you deal with is cracks in pool tables, and cheese-and-crackers."

But what about her roommate's new information, perhaps reinforcing the team's suspicion? Fortunately, in outreach work, there is a familiar expedient, always ready-to-hand: make another home visit (Section "The Pathways Model"). So, I met with her four times in that month, checking out every parameter I could think of. Her weight continued to fluctuate, mostly downwards, but she described herself as feeling "balanced." In spite of her acknowledging having discontinued her medication for the previous three months, she did not show disorganized thinking. She explained that her motive for calling the police had been a concern that her roommate was no longer working and not providing her with sufficient financial support. She engaged reasonably in a discussion about finding another medication that would not cause her to gain weight. Significantly, having discontinued art group, she agreed to return to it on a regular basis.

Taking all this into account, I stayed the course, and indeed, this crisis passed. But things were far from over, and the next time that her roommate and the team voiced their concerns, they were on point, and it was I who was off it.

Over the course of the next year, we managed to resolve these two issues. Regarding medication, she agreed to try antipsychotics not usually associated with weight gain. The first, Geodon (=ziprasidone), caused her to "fall out," a reaction I had never heard reported for this medication before, but she immediately agreed to try a second, Abilify (=aripiprazole), which she "loved" and took faithfully thereafter. Out of either prescience or some undefined sense of something metabolically wrong with herself, associated with her continuing weight loss, she requested multivitamins and calcium, which I had no hesitation about providing. Last on the topic of her medications was her request to continue taking one dose or another of Benadryl to help with sleep—a notably unlikely choice for anyone seeking to abuse mind-altering substances, which it certainly was not. Regarding the arrangement with her roommate, she agreed to have him continue living in her two-bedroom apartment, when he agreed to a $120/month increment in his payment to her, but her vacillation continued until her unrecognized general health issue provided a tactful exit from that relationship, indirectly allowing her to pursue her preference for a smaller one for herself alone.

Regarding the third issue, work, she continued to consider various jobs she had managed in the past, including hair-restorer, school security-guard, and assistant at an animal shelter, requesting support from the team's employment counselor to sort it out, though she took no definite steps.

The only remaining cloud, as the holiday season in 2006 approached, was her description of having "drifted apart" from her two children and from her mother, whom she had never spoken of previously. I offered to write a letter to her then 13-year-old daughter in Las Vegas, suggesting that she send her mother a Christmas card, and I did so, but no reply was forthcoming from her daughter. Her sadness was palpable, and it only grew.

New Issue; Course of Treatment

Not far into our third year of meetings, her behavior began to deteriorate noticeably. She became more private, requesting that I meet her outside the local post office, rather than at her apartment. After one meeting there, she failed to show up for a second one. When I was unable to locate her and called her roommate for an update, he told me she had taken herself off to the local women's shelter. For the first time I was worried about her. When I arrived there, she had already left. A counselor told me she had shown difficulty sleeping and did not appear to have any medication with her. When I finally caught up with her, the next week, she appeared distracted. She asked for a cup of coffee, which I provided, only to watch her let it grow cold, as was not her custom. Now I entertained a reasonable, but, as it turned out, inaccurate, diagnosis of major depression, manifested by her anorexia and insomnia, thinking it might have been brought on by her daughter's continuing estrangement. I offered to take her to a hospital, but she declined.

I next caught up with her on an in-patient ward at King's County Hospital. She had taken herself there, not long after our last visit, having imagined that she was suffering from some sort of psychiatric illness but having no idea what it was. She had informed the admitting psychiatrist of her ongoing treatment with me, and he, in turn, had charged a young psychiatric resident with giving me a call, ostensibly to provide his team with her background and psychiatric history. I gave them my detailed account of all our interactions over the previous two years and of my diagnosis of an extreme personality style. In response, the resident first graciously thanked me for having come and then, to my surprise and considerable chagrin, tactfully informed me that she had been screened with blood tests on admission and found to be suffering from severe hyperthyroidism. Further, he explained that, from the start of her stay, two weeks previously, she had been prescribed thyroid-suppressing medication, Tapazole (=methimazole) and was responding well clinically, to the point of resuming normal sleep and appetite; that the laboratory values reflecting her condition were showing considerable improvement; and that she would be ready for discharge shortly. Moreover, her social worker there reported her to be cooperative and well-related. What could I possibly add to that, if I had been able to rediscover my tongue?

Duly chastened and subdued, I assumed that these hospital psychiatrists had not only hit the mark but also had fixed the problem. I was greatly mistaken about the second of these. The treatment, as it turned out, had only just begun. For starters, where was she to go for follow-up care, once she left the hospital? I kept in touch with her treating psychiatrist there for a couple of months, slowly adjusting to the new reality of her condition. Then I phoned our local Medicaid clinic's primary care physician, who examined her and suggested she be hospitalized on a general medical unit, because her thyroid gland had by then increased noticeably in size. Pamela noted at the time that she "had a lightbulb in the neck," but she had had enough of institutional care after King's County and refused it.

I knew I needed some guidance, fast. I called up the local hospital in Jamaica to find out about its endocrinology clinic, and this turned out to be our destination more than a dozen times over the ensuing three and half years. Fortunately, it met on Wednesdays, one of my two days at Pathways, and even more fortunately, we fell upon a seasoned, welcoming endocrinologist of my vintage, Narinder Kukar, who was to become my unofficial mentor and team-extender. Just as my relationship with Pamela was finding a focus, so he and I began a relationship that was to ripen, as he patiently introduced me to the management of her complex condition.

In retrospect, the dramatic fluctuations in her weight during our second year of working together were probably due to her insidious, fluctuating thyroid condition, rather than to the reduction or change in her medication. That I had had the gratifying experience 40 years earlier, as a senior medical student, of making a new diagnosis of hyperthyroidism on a medical clinic patient, only to fail to recognize its signs and symptoms in Pamela's case, was just a further irony.

On the other hand, dealing with a combined psychiatric/general medical condition was just where I wanted to be. Pamela was presenting Kukar and me with a first-hand opportunity to learn what integrated care meant, day by day and over time. There was no more denying what was happening. From then on, he provided the guidance, while I filled in the gaps. Because she would not let the clinic phlebotomist do so, I took blood samples from her, so that the results of laboratory tests he ordered would be available for our next visit with him. I ensured that she received the medications he prescribed and followed up on her use of them. I scheduled her follow-up appointments and brought her to the clinic, rescheduling them when she skipped out. In the course of the next three and half years I got to know the receptionists and nurses at that clinic quite well, and without their forbearance and flexibility, the management of her condition would have been impossible. Specifically, that meant they would repeatedly work her into Kukar's morning schedule any time we would show up, waiving the usual requirement for a scheduled appointment.

Pamela was, of course, as fascinated by the changes in her condition, and as gratified by the improvements as I was, but she had her own priorities, including that her condition was only one of the issues that demanded her attention. Not even her earlier observation about the "lightbulb in the neck" made it her first priority. That was not Kukar's problem, but it was certainly mine. He diagnosed her with Grave's Disease, obtained her consent—which she proudly provided—to show her off to his residents, and predicted that she might get through the whole episode just by taking thyroid-suppressant medication.

But this was not to be. Instead, over the course of the next year, the laboratory values reflecting the progress of her thyroid disease failed to improve. She dropped to 20 lb below her usual weight, and she developed exophthalmos, the condition of protuberant eyeballs that are classic signs of Grave's Disease. Kukar concluded that it was time to move on: if she wanted to avoid surgery, she would need treatment with radioactive iodine to shrink her gland. Whether these developments resulted from taking her Tapazole inconsistently or not was beside the point. The only hitch was that the new treatment he was prescribing was not provided at Jamaica Hospital, so she and I would have to drive for 45 min each way across Queens to Jamaica's sister hospital, Brookdale.

On receipt of his recommendation, Pamela was quite unfazed, and surely, she had endured worse. She would accept being injected with radioactive iodine, but, as for what she called "snip, snip,"—i.e., surgery—that was a no-go. She must have had some hesitation, even over the prescribed treatment, because it took me three tries, over the course of three months, to collect her and get her there for her first visit. What may have tipped the balance and brought on her cheerful anticipation was a fortunate coincidence that occurred just at that moment: a telephone call from her daughter in Las Vegas, the only one she was to receive during our six years together. Thereafter, the treatment proceeded smoothly with her full cooperation over the course of several visits in the next month. But whether she followed the nuclear radiologist's injunction against coming within six feet of young children or pregnant women for the month after receiving the therapeutic dose of radioactive iodine, only Pamela knows.

Improvement in Both Systemic and Psychological Health

Perhaps she decided that she had paid enough attention to her health and was back to the central issues in her life, which were her part-time work and her absent children. For six months she eluded my efforts to get her back to Kukar for a follow-up visit. During that time, I will admit to becoming exasperated more than once. It seemed as if we had come so far, and now we were about to let success slip away. I went so far as to insist that she get herself to his clinic and then phone me to join her there, but she made it clear that was not going to happen, stating, "If they (meaning, me) want me to see Kukar, they have to call me night and day to make a sale." I settled down and resumed taking her, even adding an open bribe after each visit, namely, an egg sandwich from the next-door delicatessen.

In the end, she and Kukar were right and my concerns proved to have been exaggerated: it did not matter what further attention she paid to her treatment, for the treatment with radioactive iodine had worked, and she was on the path back to health. As for my relationship with him, he had come to know of my interest in short stories (Section "My View of How These Patients Change") and had recommended I take a look at the ancient Hindu folk tales he recalled from his youth, entitled the "Panchatantra." We had clearly been destined to wind up on the same team.

My motives in pursuing the management of her prolonged episode of hyperthyroidism were on several levels. First, there was no way I could abandon this lively and loyal woman, who had gratifyingly remained true to my psychiatric diagnosis—yes, we psychiatrists do care about a thing like that—and to the treatment for her systemic illness, no matter how much her personality style tested me. Clearly, the consequences would have been costly not only for her but also for the healthcare system: I will leave the details to your imagination. Second, I was curious to learn about the treatment of a condition that was unfamiliar to me, in spite of my brief, earlier experience. And third, I enjoyed the collaboration with the kindly medical specialist, who had such a clear idea of how to proceed—so much easier to follow than the conditions I dealt with in my usual work. So, I suppose that Pamela and I were both learning and both curious as to how things would turn out.

There were still some ups and downs in the course of her recovery: at one point it appeared she would need another course of radioactive iodine; at another, it was important to check that her protuberant eyes had not been injured by their being thus exposed. However, in the end things proceeded smoothly: her thyroid gland shrank back to almost normal size, and her bulging eyes receded somewhat. Her weight continued to fluctuate and then settled down to what it had been before the episode began. Her laboratory results showed that there was enough normally functioning tissue left to keep her from needing a thyroid supplement in the future.

Throughout this period of her early to mid-40s, Pamela had been engaged in making the transition from some frightening and painful prior experiences to a quieter and steadier, if lonelier, life. She wore her heart on her sleeve, or rather, all over her body, in her clothing, her body piercings, and her colorful way of speaking. She revealed it in her drawings. When she was with me (at first I wrote "with you," using her way of speaking), she was fully engaged, in her own, unforgettably unique way. When she was away from me (I just did the same thing again), it was another story, and obviously, I did not know when she would choose to turn up; indeed, it was better not to let my expectations get too high. It was just that she was balancing her options in both situations, and she let me know not to push her. Her roommate had once put it that, "She was never going to do anything crazy," and indeed, her judgment about her needs turned out to be quite good, including her judgment of people at the current stage of her life. Still, she was not going to accept recommendations on faith alone: they had to make sense in her terms. Her goals were modest ones, and she never wavered in her pursuit of them. Her main disappointment was in not being able to reestablish contact with her two children, for whom she felt so deeply and whose rejection she could not comprehend.

More important to her, once her hyperthyroidism cooled down, was that she returned to a focus on her personal goals. She chose ultimately to resume taking Abilify for her chronic anxiety, which she had discontinued while ill, not inappropriately. She returned to more or less consistent work as part-time assistant in a stationery store, asking sometimes that I meet her outside it, now as a sign of her health, rather than of a need for privacy, as she had, three years earlier, when she was becoming ill. She was pleased to be invited to attend a family reunion, following her grandmother's death, though, tellingly, she was shaken by meeting a niece's boyfriend, who had suffered an accident affecting his eyesight. Her son, living only in the next borough of New York City, had not contacted her in the previous two years, and her daughter had phoned only once. I supposed that sadness was behind the new appearance, one day, of tear-drop tattoos running from her eye down one side of her cheek. "Oh, those," she explained, in response to my inquiry, "Those are only raindrops."

She never did manage to organize her belongings in her apartment, which continued to resemble more of a nest, but instead insisted she would manage it better, once she moved to her third apartment, this time in Manhattan, "where you (i.e., I) grew up," and where she had always aspired to return. Her discussions of that prospect were quite realistic. She acknowledged the risk in moving further from the team's office and thus in making it harder to access support, but she assured me and herself that, "Your hands are not neuroses (i.e., I don't have to call for help each time a problem arises). You don't call unless it's an emergency." As we had begun, so we ended, with her wishing me well in my retirement but admonishing me to "be careful."

I was quite aware, all along, that my level of personal investment would not necessarily be the choice for other practitioners in my place. Perhaps, Pamela could have been convinced to work out her systemic health problem even more efficiently through another approach, such as agreeing to a short hospitalization. But in following her preferences as to how to proceed, she and I had learned some things about each other and about ourselves. In the end the successful outcome speaks for itself. I believe she had the satisfaction of building confidence in her own choices, something she would need to draw on in the future, even as her modest plans for improving the quality of her life were materializing.

Post-script

Following the closing of Pathways' operations in New York, she was reassigned to the Jamaica, Queens, team of the Post-graduate Center for Mental Health, who provided me with her telephone contact information. When I called, she agreed immediately to meet me and showed up at our appointed time, back on a familiar street corner. She was dressed, groomed, and decorated as before. She explained that she had indeed moved to an apartment in Manhattan, as she had planned, had attended a Pathways office nearby, and had resumed her drawing sessions with

Rachel Romero, who worked at that site, as well; however, for vague reasons she had lost it after a year and had moved back to one in Jamaica, though she hoped to return to Manhattan again, some day. She had found new, part-time work as a ticket-seller at a theater on the Upper West Side.

She had not required or taken any medication for anxiety in some time, causing me to wonder whether that symptom might not have been due to the early stages of hyperthyroidism, when I first met her, rather than to difficulties around her unique personality style, as I had assumed it to be. On the other hand, as a result of checking periodically with her primary care physician at the Medicaid clinic around the corner from the original Pathways office in Jamaica, she was found to need and was faithfully taking a small dose of a thyroid-replacement medication. Furthermore, in terms of health-management, she had undergone tooth extractions and bridge construction that had required multiple visits to her dentist. She was pleased with the result. I took this as evidence of her having learned to take better care of herself through the extended process of managing her hyperthyroidism, and I told her so.

Sadly, the estrangement from her children persisted: she had seen her son only once and had received no further communication from her daughter. Her mother, though still living, was now in an extended care facility and quite debilitated. "You're just for yourself," was how she put it.

I offered her a copy of the narrative I had written, and when she hesitated, I asked if she would prefer I read it aloud to her. She assented, so I began. After the first couple of pages, she indicated that she had heard enough, that she was quite pleased, and that she requested only one small change: she preferred that I keep her first name but change the initial of her last name to "P," for "Piggybank." So that is the initial you see.

Chapter 4
Bernardo H.

This story does not end well. It follows a back-and-forth pattern that made it continually difficult to gauge whether my patient was recovering. There were several points at which he seemed about to turn a corner. Certainly, he did have an idea of what he wanted his life to look like. But in the end, his fears, as well-grounded in his experiences as they might have been, kept him from taking charge of his life and maintaining it as he intended. Still, things might just as well have turned out much more favorably.

Personal and Psychiatric History

Bernardo H., a Latino man, was 53 when we met, 57 at the end. He was a proud man. He noted that his birthday, January 7, coincided in some years with the Feast of the Epiphany, emphasizing that the Three Kings recognized the baby Jesus' divinity on that day. A casual conversation would reveal that he was quite bright, without being overbearing, and that he was conversant with both historical issues and current political events. He was an open, credible, and grateful patient, even though he often complained of being misunderstood and wronged.

His early life had been a challenge for uncommon reasons, but in those days he was up to it. When he was seven, his father, a World War II veteran, adopted a Jamaican girl of five, whom he outspokenly preferred over Bernardo, and he took out his anger as a youngster by frequently getting into fights, but he never let them derail his schoolwork, where he was doing well. When he was forced to miss a year of school between age seven and eight because of an episode of tuberculosis, he managed by being an avid reader to keep up well enough to resume school with the rest of his classmates without having to drop back a year. At 18, after having dropped out of high school and having worked for 2 years at an art gallery, he "fell out" with his boss, but he soon went on to find work in record stores for nearly a decade. There he would sometimes run into celebrities from the pop music world and "felt part of

© Springer International Publishing Switzerland 2016
W. Tucker, *Narratives of Recovery from Serious Mental Illness*,
DOI 10.1007/978-3-319-33727-2_4

the scene." This was the fondest period of his life, because it showed how his intellectual gifts and interpersonal skills made him resilient and productive, up to the point that his disability supervened. We will come back to his view of it toward the end of the story.

Significant family at the time of our meetings included only a younger brother, who had served in Viet Nam, who now worked as a repairman for a technology company, and who played a significant part in the background of the central issue in this story, though there was no ongoing contact between them. He described his mother's family as "lower-middle-class Puerto Ricans" and as "warm and inviting," in contrast to his father's, who were "snobbish," but whatever they did for or to him when he was growing up, none of them figured in this story either. Given that he was quite personable and engaged with neighborhood acquaintances and, somewhat later, with employers who cared about him, I should have been more attuned to his isolation from family and the absence of close friends.

The origin of the symptoms that precipitated his first psychiatric hospitalization remained obscure. At age 27, while he was in the middle of a handball game, he suddenly began hearing in his head the Spanish words to a song. They were accompanied by "children's voices—not scary or saying anything negative—and visions, like a TV screen." If I had been paying attention to the report of the visual hallucinations, I might have inquired about the possibility of the context of drug or alcohol use. However, I failed to do so.

Whatever the nature of his illness, it was severe enough to derail his life completely. Thereafter, he "struggled" for two decades, accumulating a string of hospitalizations for episodes like the first, so that, by his mid-40s, he found himself homeless. He lived in a shelter for a month and a half, before being assigned one of Pathways' apartments, which he was to occupy until we met, 6 years later. The hospitalization that was to be his last had occurred in 2005, just before we met.

Since he greeted me at our first meeting with an account of his conviction that people he saw on the street were talking about him, I assumed he might indeed deserve the diagnosis of a delusional illness, even though he did not report having experienced any cognitive or mood symptoms at all; indeed, his thinking was quite logical around all subjects but one. This assumption turned out to be incorrect, or rather, only secondary like Gary's (Chap. 2), in view of the overwhelming evidence of something else that he presented repeatedly during our encounters over the ensuing four and one-half years. And he never again mentioned that people on the street were talking about him.

Treatment Issues

When we first met, he tried to cast his life in a favorable light, with only a hint of sadness that his earlier life had been disrupted. He talked of enjoying good food and concerts, when he could afford them. He ascribed his way of interpreting other people's actions to his "analytical mind—not paranoia;" either way, the Haldol he was taking regularly kept him "focused." He was thinking about writing a play about mental illness and Pathways' supportive role. He kept himself busy writing music and shopping for stylish but inexpensive clothes for the approaching summer. Overall, he felt he was "doing well other than financially."

But it soon emerged that he was dissatisfied and frustrated with almost everything he confronted: high-cost-but-low-quality medical care, inconsistencies in the social security system, the departure from Pathways of an admired team leader, faithless women, aggressive neighborhood "punks," and worst of all, the many people who tried constantly to criticize and belittle him. That last, I realized later, was meant as a caution, lest I be included among them.

Furthermore, there were two immediate problems on his mind. One was persistent pain in his left knee, the result of having been struck by an automobile, a year previously, requiring tendon repair at the Hospital for Special Surgery immediately following the accident, and necessitating his sporting a fancy, carved-wood cane with a sharp tip, that may have come in handy for other things besides walking. The other was his concern about having Hepatitis C infection, though he assured us both that a physician at the Elmhurst clinic had told him that his was not "full-blown" and therefore did not yet need treatment. This was eventually to become our most frequent topic of discussion. He never managed to resolve either problem.

Nevertheless, for the next 2 years, he remained fairly stable. I heard him deliver a kind and appropriate eulogy for a deceased fellow-client of Pathways. At the beginning of a new year and in celebration of his birthday, he landed a part-time job at a neighborhood shoe store, where he enjoyed chatting with customers, several of whom were acquaintances. He maintained his appearance. I felt no pressure to challenge his expressed preference that we stick to world political and cultural events in our meetings and not probe too deeply into troubling issues, such as his health.

A pattern emerged whereby he would introduce an aspect of one of these issues and his plan for addressing it, only to drop the subject or announce at the next visit that he was postponing the intervention a bit longer. At some point in the cycle I would offer to join forces with him to achieve the result that he, after all, had expressed a desire for. Then, if I persisted, he would let me know, in no uncertain terms, that I was "pressuring" him, and that he would prefer to move back to a more impersonal subject. This tacit agreement between us on how to proceed worked for us—or rather, in fact, failed us—because there would frequently be an indication that he was making some progress, however slight, even if we had agreed to avoid his immediate problems.

There were many such examples. First, here is what happened with his knee pain. Having mentioned at our first meeting that he had scheduled an appointment the next month at the Hospital for Special Surgery for evaluation of whether he required secondary repair, he proceeded to cancel the appointment repeatedly with the excuse that the pain was subsiding, thus bringing about "a turning point in [his] life;" or that he did not want to undergo surgery over the summer, because he wanted to enjoy it, or over the fall, because the surgeons would then be focused on sports injuries; or, finally, that "they could experiment on someone else." Later, he preferred taking analgesic medication for the knee pain, including codeine, which the physician at Elmhurst used to prescribe, but whom he had stopped seeing. He requested it from me, and I provided it for a few months, even while recognizing that I was colluding with his avoidance of dealing definitively with the problem.

The same pattern characterized the management of his finances. In the beginning, he asked me a few times for a monthly prescription for Viagra, only later explaining that he had not had sexual relations in a decade, because he feared disease, and because he did not want to pass on his Hepatitis C, and because a woman he cared for had betrayed him and broken his heart. "Does that mean I'm a faggot?" he asked, obviously in pain over many issues. So, presumably, he was selling the tablets for a small profit to spend on those cherished restaurant meals and concerts. But this was only an incidental source of income. He had received a settlement of $9,500 from the insurance company of the driver whose car had struck him the year before we met. Then it turned out that, because of that sum, he had become ineligible for Supplemental Security Income, leading him to become short of funds, as soon as he had run through the settlement money. With the loss of SSI came the loss of Medicaid. Pathways staked him to a loan, and his lawyer managed to get him reinstated back into SSI and Medicaid, but by then he had gone through a significant part of an additional $3000 that SSI had provided to replace the payments he had missed.

Obstacles to Improvement

More important than either of these issues in the end was that his ineligibility for Medicaid helped provide an excuse for postponing his addressing his hepatitis. When he was reinstated, he expressed a preference for signing up at the clinic he knew to be associated with my home-base, Columbia Presbyterian Medical Center. It seemed he felt a bond with me, and I thought that might help reduce his anxiety, which, I assumed, arose from having heard reports of the imposing side effects of Interferon, then the standard treatment for that infection. Then, however, he brought up another, ultimately insurmountable basis for that anxiety. He reported that his younger brother had contracted the same infection during his tour of duty in Viet Nam; that it had destroyed his liver, necessitating a liver transplant; and that he had required a course of Interferon thereafter to clear the lingering infection. This course of treatment apparently raised such a frightening specter that Bernardo preferred to forgo evaluation altogether. He hinted as much, when he expressed his fear that Interferon was "like chemotherapy." The pattern of the fluctuations around all these highly fraught subjects appears, in retrospect, like an extended conversation, in which he slowly spun out a chain of related thoughts to me, ones that he juggled constantly in his mind but could not face altogether.

At what might have become a turning point, he refused my offer to meet him at Columbia and accompany him to the clinic there. He could not have failed to be aware of what was happening to him, because he repeatedly attributed his "chronic fatigue" to his diseased liver, even while insisting it was "not yet inflamed," based on its not being "tender." Again and again, he refused to let me draw a blood sample to find out what treatment, if any, he might require.

By now you will probably have surmised that the real issue underlying all of the above inconsistencies was his almost daily consumption of large amounts of alcohol. This was the most likely cause of his two decades of what he called "struggle," prior to his finding what he called his "grounding" at Pathways. There had been some polysubstance abuse in the past, but this was no longer part of the picture. It was drinking, pure and simple. My efforts to warn him, regularly, for more than 2 years, that the combination of alcohol and Hepatitis C was highly dangerous, must only have frightened him further; after all, he knew from his brother's experience, as well as I did, just what the consequences could be. He summed up the situation by acknowledging that "liver transplant is out of the question for me, because they're not going to give it to someone who's drinking."

It was clear enough what he was doing, because the signs of his drinking were obvious: he would routinely fail to remove his sunglasses; his brow would sweat profusely, no matter what the season; and he often had alcohol on his breath. Nor did he deny his habit; on the contrary, he would defend it vociferously, stating variously that life without alcohol was boring, or that he consumed only small quantities, or that "nobody's perfect."

The problem with our tacit agreement not to pursue this troubling issue was that it could break down in the face of repeated signs of the many problems it was causing him, and then both of us would have to scramble. That is precisely what began to happen, 2 years into our meetings.

The first indication we got was that several of our team members reported seeing him inebriated on his job. They asked him to attend a meeting with all of us, which clearly unsettled him. When we next met, he complained that no one at the meeting had addressed him directly but me. He manifested a hand tremor for the first time, but he attributed it to the haloperidol he had been taking without complaint for the previous 2 years. He requested changing it to Mellaril (=thioridazine), an antipsychotic which was less likely to cause tremors, and which he had taken before coming to Pathways. Then he promptly lost the new prescription I gave him. He also reported having lost eligibility for food stamps.

Shortly thereafter, the team announced it would make a visit to his apartment, in response to complaints from his superintendent, to clean out what he called his "accumulated trash." I went along, but I was not prepared for the shock I received when we walked in. He acknowledged later that it must have appeared "pretty rough—pretty macho," an understatement to describe the piles of paper and plastic bags of trash and garbage I noted lined up along three walls, with debris scattered about the center of the room. The entire floor was bare, the carpet having been rolled up against the fourth wall. It looked as if the occupant must be on the verge of departing, though he was not. What was most disturbing was that he did not appear to be disturbed, but rather, only matter-of-factly playing the host. Later, he complained of having felt "criticized" at the confrontation. He was, after all, a man who prided himself on dressing and looking well, no matter how tight his budget, and the dilapidated appearance of his apartment must have been humiliating to him.

Efforts at Improvement

He pulled himself together once more and added a second a part-time job, distributing flyers for a hair salon. I asked whether he thought any aspect of his own behavior would interfere with his new job. "No," he replied, "the future is in my hands. I don't have it so bad, compared to brain-damaged Iraq War vets." As before, he was mostly preoccupied with various plans for intellectual exercises. One was to start a discussion group around experiences of 9/11 for fellow-clients. Another was to write about homelessness, but as fiction rather than as his own experiences.

When I learned from his boss that his drinking presented a problem, I could not refrain from passing on the boss's concern and pointing out that consuming alcohol was quite dangerous, given his hepatitis. "You're putting me down," he replied, and again we changed the subject. I must have been frustrated to have gone along with him that time, because my notes for this meeting were sprinkled with pejorative labels from the list of the various personality disorders I had just decided were causing him to deny the obvious.

These exchanges continued for another year. No amount of reassurance that the first step was only to get an evaluation, and that he could decide about treatments afterwards, would suffice to get him started. The drinking continued. The team was increasingly concerned and prescribed more frequent visits, to little effect. "I'm at the borderline between ecstasy and depression," he announced. "I'm going to try making a start in the new year about stopping drinking." When it came and went, he promised, "Okay, I'll start in March." He was concerned that a fellow-client he considered a friend had just died of complications of diabetes. By the summer he had lost 15 lb and was becoming frightened. Finally, in December, he announced, "I should stop fooling myself and get checked."

Once again, so much time had elapsed, and so many exchanges had ended in painful stalemates, that I never came to a point of taking definitive action.

My next and, as it turned out, last approach was to invite him to discuss a short story with me, an intervention I had found useful in situations of impasse with numerous private patients in the past (Section "My View of How These Patients Change"). I suggested one by Machiavelli, called "Belfagor: Story of the Devil Who Took a Wife," which concerns the character's effort to prove that it is women who cause men to incur damnation. Bernardo replied that he was not familiar with that particular story, but that he had read *The Prince* and knew Machiavelli "wrote about power." When we finally got around to discussing it, another 6 months later, he appeared quite moved, saying it reminded him, somehow, of the songs he liked in happier days during his adolescence, when he was working in the record store. Neither of us knew for sure what was coming, but both of us were very worried.

When we met next, he reported having given up drinking in the evenings, not because he wanted to try to improve his health, but because he had lost his job. Fear of loss of employment is the only motivation that, statistically, has an immediate impact on drinking behavior, but his boss had taken the further step of firing him.

Would he have agreed to give Bernardo another chance if I had asked him to? Things were now happening too fast. As a result of suddenly discontinuing drinking, Bernardo now suffered from terrible insomnia and requested a sleep medication. To me this was a convincing detail in support of the validity of his report. So desperate was he over this new development that he willingly accepted trazadone, which is non-habit-forming, and which he had refused in the past. Indeed, his guard was down, and he at last acknowledged some of the chaos in his life.

Success or Failure?

Three weeks later, I received a call from the Queens Medical Examiner's office, informing me that the autopsy performed on the body found in Bernardo's apartment showed death from liver failure, a consequence of the cirrhosis he must have been developing all along. The Assistant Examiner, whom I went to see there, requested help in identifying the badly decomposed body, which had been determined to have lain more than a week before being discovered. She wanted to be able to make a positive identification, so that he could be interred with a proper headstone, rather than in an unmarked grave. Though protocol precluded my viewing the body directly, she presented me with a picture, but the face was unrecognizable. Based on her extensive experience in making identifications, she inquired whether there had not been an x-ray, perhaps, that would coincide with one her office had taken of the body, showing the distinctive fracture-line in a rib that she had noticed. I recalled Bernardo's having told me of having been hospitalized for a bout of severe bronchitis, a decade before we met, and that hospital's records department, which I contacted, was indeed able to produce the required evidence: a chest x-ray with the same distinctive feature in one of the ribs.

This process had required several return visits to the ME's office, during which it felt as if I were bringing closure to a relationship that had eluded me. I looked back over a series of occasions, even if initially out of ignorance, when I had colluded with his requests for Viagra prescriptions and thus allowed him his version of how we were to proceed; when he found part-time work in a shoe store and was enjoying friendly social contact and, once again, having some small personal pleasure on his own terms; when he changed his Medicaid coverage to a type that was accepted at the hospital where I was affiliated, in preparation for undergoing an evaluation he trusted; when, at least in my mind, we shared the enjoyment of a short story. On those occasions I had felt that we were coming closer to a meeting of the minds, and that he might still save himself. There was not that far remaining for him to go.

The only positive effect of this small gap was that he continued to live his life on his own terms to the end, even to the point that he realized, in both senses of the word, the validity his own, long-standing fears—the ones that finally prevented his taking hold of his health and his life. It would have been more satisfying during these few weeks, to have enlisted the support of his brother, but he had lost his job and had moved from the only address we had on file, so I did not manage to contact him. I felt I had done what I could for Bernardo, given the extent of my limited understanding. But I will always wonder whether I might have approached him differently, early on, and thus, whether he might not have overcome his fears and thus, faced his drinking and fatal self-neglect. Most people afflicted with significant substance abuse require structure to support their efforts to quit—Gary (Chap. 2) is an excellent example, but whereas he recognized this need and sought it out, Bernardo never got that far.

Right now, if you have not done so already, you must be wondering how this can be considered a narrative of recovery. Bernardo claimed he was satisfied with his lifestyle, up until the point when he lost his job, abruptly stopped drinking, and experienced withdrawal symptoms; in fact, he had defended his right to live as he was doing all along. He had friends, part-time work, and at least modest pleasures, such as dining out and dressing nicely. This was the life he wanted for himself. So, what had prevented him from taking care of his health—only one more small step, and one that would have allowed him to keep on going as he chose? Why had he needed to lose his job, in order to be convinced to stop drinking?

You may insist that we never know for sure that even when someone in retrospect attributes her/his recovery from substance abuse to a particular experience, she/he may only be telling a story to explain a change that has many antecedents, known and unknown. Surely that is true in general. But in this specific case I had a different opinion. He was, after all, a highly intelligent man, and he had not so damaged his critical faculties with drink as to be unable to imagine where he was heading. In fact his ability to do so was itself the problem. I felt he was terribly frightened of having to endure the pain his brother had gone through to address the same condition, and furthermore, Bernardo was aware that he would not be eligible for it, even if he had chosen to proceed. Instead, he kept putting off the decision to stop drinking and go through the abstinence period required of potential transplant candidates. Self-medication with alcohol for his resultant anxiety sealed the deal. Would he have had a different outcome, if I had figured this out when he first told me, 4 years earlier, of his brother's experience and its impact on his thinking? I never got to find out.

Post-script

All my efforts to reach Bernardo's only known relative, his younger brother, failed. I got as far as a street address and telephone number in Greer, SC, to which he had moved, after losing his job in Connecticut, but the number had been disconnected without further information. Bernardo had told me of two older brothers but not their names, so I could not trace them. I have therefore changed his first name and initial, to protect his anonymity.

Chapter 5
Victoria N.

This is a complicated story, partly because of the stepwise revelation of the main clinical problem, and partly because of the interactions with several important family members and, ultimately, of the patient's need for crucial guidance and services from an outside agency. Even in retrospect it does not seem to me that clues were missed along the way that might have been recognized even sooner; rather, both the patient and I only gradually identified the main issue, as it emerged over time. Progress toward recovery, once it began, was quite steady overall, though there was some back-and-forth in mood and behavior. As with the previous narratives, such a pattern of gradual recognition is probably not rare, so long as the psychiatrist is open to its being there and willing to revise both diagnosis and approach as s/he goes along, rather than being bound either by her/his own initial clinical assumptions or by the exigencies of the electronic record, whose demand for a definitive diagnosis at the time of initial encounter is indelible and resistant to updating.

First Impressions

Victoria N. appeared to be a somewhat youngish but otherwise typical 19-year-old adolescent girl when I first met her, 3 months into my tenure at Pathways. She had a high school diploma and some work experience as a home health aide but lacked any real direction in her life or even real enthusiasms, beyond dancing and pop music. She had arrived on Pathways' doorstep after losing her job, and she was living in one of our houses along with three other female clients. It was not even so clear to me, at first, how much time she was spending lounging around in bed each day. What struck me was how absolutely comfortable she was having a much older, male psychiatrist visit her regularly in her bedroom. As there was no free chair, I had to choose between standing up and sitting on the edge of her bed, where she lay stretched out under the sheets. I saw her a dozen times in our first half-year, which

© Springer International Publishing Switzerland 2016
W. Tucker, *Narratives of Recovery from Serious Mental Illness*,
DOI 10.1007/978-3-319-33727-2_5

must have been a record frequency of visits for me. All of this might have made me wonder what was going on, but it was probably just as well that it did not, because I would then have gotten ahead of her story.

Her symptom presentation was classic for schizophrenia: she described herself as "dead, lost, alone, and miserable"; she was certain that others could read her thoughts (=thought broadcasting); and she reported that she was unable to concentrate, confused about her identity, and highly ambivalent. She had been prescribed a non-sedating, non-weight-augmenting antipsychotic, Geodon (=ziprasidone), but had discontinued it after a single dose, "because it made my feet hurt"—an unlikely side-effect, to say the least. Her clothes were filthy, and her hair, unkempt. On a recent visit to a dentist's office concerning a wisdom tooth extraction, the receptionist's negative reaction to her manner and appearance made her "wish [she] wouldn't think at all." The last time she had felt well was two months previously, on a visit to a half-sister in Arizona.

Perhaps you can guess the state of her room. Clothes were strewn all about, spilling out of the drawers of the bureau and of a trunk. There were a couple of colorful posters on the wall and a dark cloth over one of the windows, whose blinds were missing. Open packages of junk food and half-empty soda cans lay everywhere on furniture, window sills, and floor. Vermin were not yet in evidence, but you could imagine them just ready to emerge. Of course, it would only be fair to wonder whether this state of disorganization was due to illness or merely to adolescence.

On my third visit, a month later, there was more bad news: first, the report of mild suicidal ideation, "I wish I weren't here"; next, and nearly as bad, the report that, during the previous week, a woman in her early 30s, whom Victoria had been pursuing romantically for a year, had stabbed her in the back and shoulder to make her desist in her pursuit. In despair she had stood outside in front her own house, taken off all her clothes, and conversed with several men who, unsurprisingly, had stopped to gawk at her. I concluded that she was psychotic and in need of closer supervision and immediate resumption of medication, if she was to avoid hospitalization.

Initial Response to Treatment

I duly instituted oral haloperidol, which she agreed, reluctantly, to try. When I returned the next day, accompanied by our team nurse, who belatedly cleaned and dressed her wounds, she seemed already somewhat improved, in terms of both affect and cognition. Though the improvement could not have been due to the medication, because she had not taken it, I was not up for chancing her further deterioration, and she accepted an injection of long-acting haloperidol this time without objection.

By her own estimation, over the ensuing 3 months she went from "60 % improved" to "80 %" to "over 80 %." In this time period she had managed to tidy her room, dress and groom herself smartly, and take visits from friends. She said the thought broadcasting had stopped. Furthermore, she began to talk of wanting to return to her former job, "Because I don't like having so much time to lie here, staring at walls." She requested I ask her grandmother for an invitation to Thanksgiving dinner, and her grandmother consented, acknowledging Victoria's improvement on all fronts.

The typical monthly schedule of visits offered in clinics where I have worked assume a regularity and stability of behavior and needs that is quite inadequate for people not yet settled in their routines, as Victoria certainly was not. Occasional extra visits, even back-to-back ones, were not unusual for me, but with her, this increased frequency was to become a pattern: we had met twice monthly, on average, over our first half-year together, and we were to continue at this rate over the ensuing year. It turned out to be a good thing that I had the flexibility to accommodate her needs.

Six months into accepting haloperidol injections, she had recovered entirely from the psychotic symptoms I was rightly or wrongly attributing to her, and she had impressed her immediate family with her improvement. Thereupon, she refused to accept further medication, asserting that she had only been "stressed out" and "depressed" before. Six months later, she was once more reported by Pathways staff to have been found walking naked in the street and was briefly hospitalized involuntarily, before being sent back to a room that was, once again, a mess.

Family History

Before I drag you into the thicket of current family expectations and demands, let me back up and provide what I understood about some of the members. These included her father, her maternal grandparents, her grandmother's boyfriend, girl-friends from high school, and her mother's current boyfriend. Her father, who remained in Jamaica, was apparently supportive and noncritical but also ineffectual, well meaning but also unreliable, making promises but not fulfilling them. She occasionally phoned him and, later on, sent him money, but never pursued intentions of flying back to visit him. Her mother had her own troubled early development. She was taken away from her own mother and raised by her father, whom Victoria's grandmother described as "a bad influence," as a way of excusing some of the mother's critical and rigid attitudes toward Victoria. Fortunately, early on, back in Jamaica, there had yet another player on the scene, namely, the grandmother's boyfriend, who took her and her mother into their house, when Victoria was still a toddler, and provided stability and tranquility that Victoria frequently recalled with pleasure.

Thus, when she asserted that she "raised [her-]self from the age of five," it emerged that the conflicts were internal, rather than imposed upon her. Keep that particular age in mind, and you will shortly see a connection that I had missed. She did not reveal what those conflicts were until the second and third years of our work together. As for the mother herself there was no doubt that she did her best to understand Victoria, but because of her traditional religious and cultural background, she had trouble understanding and accepting what she sensed was unfolding. Other players include, of course, the grandmother, who was there from the beginning. She had brought Victoria and her mother from the island of Jamaica to The Bronx, when Victoria was a young adolescent, and had remained close-by as a generally positive influence up to the present. There were also two girlfriends she had known since high school and for whose young children she sometimes babysat. Finally, there was her mother's boyfriend, whom you will meet shortly. There was thus a network much richer than that of most of our Pathways clients for her to draw on, and she did just that. You may also consider that rich network a sign of health, and if so, I would agree with those of you who might be questioning my initial diagnosis

Gender Issue(s)

However, shortly before the new developments, she had responded to my inquiry about her not having resumed work, which she had considered crucial to her mental health, with an abrupt revelation, namely, that she was horribly conflicted over being gay. I had not considered this possibility at all, and, as it turned out, she did not understand its dimensions fully, either. "It's disgusting, unnatural, and unfair," she asserted, adding that, since Pathways' staff could not help her with it, she only wanted to be left alone. "My mind is clear—too clear. I keep my clothes on, I don't think people are reading my mind, and I'm eating and sleeping okay. My only problem is that I prefer women sexually." Needless to say, her mother was urgently requesting a meeting, only to be told there by Victoria that "I knew I liked women since I was five!" Her mother responded first by inquiring about the utility of hormone treatments to change her thinking but then settled for taking her to a hair salon for a beauty treatment.

That revelation, which was not to be the last one, may have precipitated a crisis for Victoria and for her mother, but it also began moving things forward again, in a direction none of us could have foreseen, namely, Victoria's first move toward acknowledging and taking charge of her own condition. In short order she agreed to accept injections again, if Pathways would arrange for her to have her own apartment. Meanwhile, she lived successively at the local YMCA and then, while her new apartment was being refurbished, with a fellow Pathways client, a man. She got herself briefly rehospitalized again for climbing out his window "without any thought of self-harm," thereafter, she resumed taking long-acting haloperidol. Six months into our second year together, she was capably managing her own apartment, cooking Jamaican specialties for friends and family, and looking for work. However, a note to myself at this time expresses skepticism that even an effective antipsychotic could be this good. So, I should not have been surprised that yet another revelation was in store.

It was another nine months before Victoria announced to me that she had just recently begun discussions with our team nurse about her desire for sex change surgery. Finally her real secret was out: the reason she had to "raise [her]-self since age five" was not merely that she realized at that age that she "preferred girls," but that she was "a boy in a girl's body." (From now on I will refer to this man with the masculine pronoun, for a man he is, indeed.) No amount of struggle over the next three-plus years ever extinguished completely the feeling that, as he put it, "It's not fair! It shouldn't have happened to me." Still, this moment marked the beginning of a transformation from which he never looked back. Henceforth he had a goal that would focus all his efforts—on work, on organizing his finances, on learning new behaviors, and on "stay[ing] out of trouble." The way to the change he desired was neither straight nor swift, but he realized that at least there was a way. A significant benefit for him from this cascade of realizations, coming from his very traditional cultural tradition, was that, as a man, he could view his preference for women as heterosexual, rather than homosexual: if one is a man, then preferring sex with women is the traditional choice.

You will not be surprised to learn that my response to his announcement was immediately to search the Internet for sites offering sex change surgery, while simultaneously presenting the little I knew of all the preliminary steps: a trial of male hormones, of cross-dressing and living as a male, and, most important of all, of returning to work and beginning to save money—a lot of it—in anticipation of someday undergoing surgery. Much earlier in my career, I had been entrusted with a large collection of records for a deceased psychiatrist's former transgender patients, who had sought clearance for sex change surgery. From that exposure I had some acquaintance with the necessary procedures, but I had little acquaintance with the details. As little as I knew of the timing and pace of the hormonal treatments, I knew even less of the process of social transformation. For example, how does a heterosexual man born a woman go about finding a heterosexual woman receptive to his advances? More generally, what does it mean to live as a man, on a trial basis, to become used to the role? Fortunately for us both, there was outside help available, as there had been around the cultural issues. A colleague from Columbia with expertise in this area told me to contact Callen-Lorde, an agency in New York City providing both information and treatment on the whole range of LGBTQ issues. It was to become our major resource.

Early Improvement

Once I had made the initial informational contacts, my role was simply to encourage him, again and again, to take his search for answers there, along with his requests for treatment. After missing one such meeting billed as "trans/partners," he complained, "I need help, looking as I do. People say, 'Hey, girl'—that's crazy, isn't it? They know you've got a woman's parts on your body. I wish I could just wake up one day and say, 'I have parts like I am.'" He was initially so skeptical and hesitant that he required being accompanied to his first visit by our team nurse. Later, he insisted that he did not want "information" but only "help," meaning hormonal treatment and access to next steps, leading to surgery. As for attending support groups tailored to his tight work schedule, he had to be convinced that they could offer valuable guidance on appropriate and successful social interactions, in order to overcome his disappointment that they did not also simultaneously provide suitable women for his affections.

I did not think that getting clearance would present an obstacle for Victor (his new name) and was not at that moment focused on throwing up any others besides those he already contemplated. Our next three and one-half years of work were directed at his goal of becoming the man on the outside whom he knew himself to be on the inside.

Along the way he shed all the symptoms I had regarded as belonging to the realm of psychopathology: clinical depression, thought broadcasting, ambivalence, poor concentration, even suicidal thinking and behaviors. In retrospect each of these symptoms could be ascribed to his confusion about aspects of his transsexuality and to conflicts with family members and with his assailant over it. It was quite dramatic how these symptoms disappeared, once the possibility of dealing openly and directly with it began to dawn upon him.

But you may also have been struck, as I certainly was, by the dramatically effective protection against depression that long-acting haloperidol somehow conferred on him. As he put it, "the medication prevents me from having bad thoughts." So, I have little doubt that most traditional practitioners would have initially found him quite ill, as I did, and they would perhaps have been just as puzzled as I was, at his insistence on continuing to receive monthly injections indefinitely, even after the issues were out in the open, his symptoms, gone.

The first issue that he clarified, once he had at last identified his transsexuality, was the nature of his symptoms. His "thought broadcasting," he explained, was limited to Renee, who was the only person he ever thought was able to read his thoughts. His initial presentation of depression, manifested especially by poor self-care, was in response to her violent rejection of his advances, as were his later overdoses of Tylenol. As for his thoughts of going out the window of a skyscraper, such as the Empire State Building, in fact, he had never even considered taking a trip to Manhattan to look it over. As for continuing to pursue his assailant, after a protracted period of rumination and ambivalence over reestablishing contact with her, he simply pointed one day to the large keloid over his left shoulder and announced, "She gave this to me, and I don't need to see her anymore." He continued to have transient thoughts of harming himself, whenever he would feel "unable to imagine working out a life that would make sense," but he never again acted upon them.

This awareness did not altogether prevent him from courting the danger of a relapse: he subsequently pursued another woman, Babette, with an outcome similar to that with Renee, when he managed to provoke Babette's boyfriend to hit him with a stick that nearly broke his arm; still, he never sank back into a prolonged period of depression. As he put it, "I was depressed when I dressed like a woman. Now I'm sad sometimes, because I still have a woman's parts and not a man's, but I know there's help out there, so I don't get really depressed."

That resilience may be attributed to the second of his favorable responses, namely, the pursuit of work on a regular basis, without the interruptions he was previously given to. When one of the home health aide agencies required him to take a written and a practical exam, I suggested he study with our team nurse and offered to help him practice taking so-called "vital signs." When one of his clients complained that he talked too much about his problematic pursuit of Babette, he sought out another client, filling in on weekends elsewhere in the meantime. At one point he even considered being an egg donor, until I suggested that the $4 K he would suddenly come into would only compromise his SSI status. It would take him another two years and other important demonstrations of his newly announced identity, before he would open a savings account where he could put aside some of the $300–$400 per week that he was earning. For another year, in spite of the beating that nearly broke his arm, he continued to expend most of his earnings on clothes for Babette. He sent his father bail money, which he needed after being jailed for breaking a man's foot. He never visited him back in Jamaica, but when he got around to calling him and telling him of his new identity, "a big burden came off my shoulders."

Cultural Issues

The third of the crucial responses that Victor's clear focus opened for him were his relations to family and their cultural issues. Here I would have been out of my depth without considerable help. Fortunately, this help was readily forthcoming from Pathways' director of family therapy training, Lascelles Black. He must have realized I needed him, when he got wind of the family having moved into Victor's apartment. What had precipitated these family meetings, which you might have thought were inevitable, given the tensions between him and his mother ever since her arrival in New York, was the loss of her fiancé's job, which meant they could no longer pay their own rent. They had initially shown up to refurbish Victor's new apartment, which they had found in disarray, attributing it to the carelessness of the male fellow client who was a frequent visitor; however, once they had succeeded in ejecting him, they moved in themselves on a full-time basis, bringing along the fiancé's adolescent son.

As noted above (Chap. 3) Pathways has no policy precluding such arrangements, as long as they are not harmful to the client, and the latter does not object. But for Victor the issue of how to manage his mother's intrusiveness without either giving in or rejecting her, now further complicated by his new identity, was by no means simple. I believe that it was Black's intervention in these two family meetings that helped resolve this issue smoothly, without the need for painful confrontation. I could not have imagined such a resolution otherwise.

Victor excused himself from our first meeting with his mother and her fiancé, saying he was scheduled to work. Perhaps because of his absence rather than in spite of it, things got off to a favorable start, with the fiancé's assertion that, if Babette's boyfriend ever threatened Victor again, "He'd have me to reckon with." Continuing in this supportive direction, both of them then asserted their belief that Victor's problem was "spiritual, not schizophrenia." When I asked his mother why, in that case, she had threatened him with hospitalization, she replied she had never intended to follow through. Urged on by her fiancé, she presented her view of Victor's new (to her) gender identity, namely, that it was the result of her having committed an indiscretion toward a rival, who retaliated by directing a "curse" at her, which "missed" her and instead "struck" her daughter. Therefore, she wanted to proceed with a religious intervention. Though not unfamiliar with this sort of explanation, I was at a loss as to how to respond in a way that would protect both Victor and his mother, now trying her best to understand the new situation. Black was at no such loss. He noted matter-of-factly that he had seen several such cases, in none of which the patient had ever given up the conviction of having been born in the wrong body, so that if she clung to the idea of subjecting Victor to a religious intervention, she could expect that it would not undo his conviction but only, as he put it, "break him." To my surprise and relief, she accepted this from him, as if it were simply a natural fact.

In spite of having promised to attend "at least one" such meeting Victor excused himself from our next family meeting with the same excuse as before. This one opened similarly, with the mother's complaints, this time about his lavishing his earnings on various women. As before, Black suggested she not get drawn into arguments about Victor's sexual preferences and lifestyle. His responses to her, it seemed to me, were effective in diffusing not only the tension between her and her son, but also her own internal conflicts about how to process the challenge her son presented: she was, after all, reflecting her traditional culture's widely held view. Her response this time was to announce that she was thinking of moving back to Wisconsin, where she had relatives, and where she would focus on raising her young daughter, Victor's half-sister.

Her fiancé had a couple of further surprises for us. First, he announced he was returning to Georgia to oversee more closely his adolescent daughter's education, out of dissatisfaction with the liberal attitude of her school principal, who tolerated talk of lesbianism. When Lascelles, never fazed, asked what he thought his daughter's response would have been, if the principal had condemned such talk, he responded without hesitation that his daughter would simply have stopped reporting such talk to him, even though it must have been the first time he had considered the principal's motives. Second, as if empathizing with Victor's dilemma, he announced that, if Victor was to be a man, "he should be a good one: upstanding, responsible, capable of protecting himself better than he does now, and above all, not chasing every girl he sees on the street." Their discomfort, and consequently, their pressure on my patient had diminished considerably.

Of course, I kept Victor informed of the interactions at those two family meetings. The third one, which did not include his mother and her fiancé, finally brought him and Black together. In their absence Victor was able to acknowledge how self-destructive it was to pursue Babette, even though, he added, "for a kiss on the cheek, I'd just keep on doing it." Feeling much less pressured, I thought, on learning the results of the two family meetings, he experienced much less ambivalence and was able to concede that he could tolerate having his mother and her fiancé stay on a bit longer with him, after all. He never raised the issue again, though it took the two of them another six months to move out and on with their own respective lives.

The fourth and most significant of the responses to his acknowledgment of transsexuality was, of course, his growing awareness of what he needed to do to transform himself, and his taking steps to make that happen. From the start he leapt to the final one, sex change surgery. In fact this step still remained far off, even at the time I left Pathways, three and one-half years after his initial announcement. Some of the steps were gradual and intermediate, such as his dress, hairstyle, and demeanor. As he grew more comfortable, he progressed from wearing drab, baggy, and androgynous clothing, to a sort of military style uniform that was at least clean and pressed, and from there, to a mannish outfit, open down the front, that could pass for stylish at a local nightclub. He topped off the clothing with a shaved head burnished with sideburns. These changes were not uniformly progressive; rather, in their back-and-forth movement they reflected not only self-image but also self-esteem and moment-to-moment shifts in mood.

Early on in this process, it was hard to guess which of the several works-in-progress he would be presenting to me at each visit, but, as time went on, his progress became unmistakable. Another concrete step that I never imagined but easily recognized as significant was his getting a Green Card to make his recently masculinized name official. How many of you would have seen that as its primary purpose? This fairly straightforward achievement brought him both pride and delight—not to mention that it removed his final excuse for delaying opening a savings account. He was pleased when his physician at Callen-Lorde noted that his voice sounded lower.

Continuing Improvement

As this transformation progressed, my role changed from physician to a combination of coach for him and interlocutor for agencies and Pathways personnel. He requested that our regular meetings be held around the corner from the apartment of one of his clients, so as not to interfere with his work schedule. Invariably they involved my administering his monthly injection, which he was not ready to forego. As he put it, "I take Haldol in the arm, to keep from getting depressed, and hormones in the thigh." You may well imagine that a team of six or more individuals, regardless of their professional training, would hold a range of views on a subject as commonly threatening as transsexuality. So it was with our team, initially. But as Victor's obvious blossoming became increasingly apparent to all of us, our hesitations tended to fade, even without the need for direct confrontation, just as Victor's parents' had under Black's gentle ministrations. Outside agencies, from Social Security to his employer, required occasional letters of verification, but they, likewise, accepted the reality I was only too ready to support.

Paradoxically, my role as coach was facilitated by my lack of relevant experience with the critical issues, which I left him to address during his gradually more frequent visits to Callen-Lorde. When he complained that breast reduction surgery was expensive, I countered that he might not need it at all, if the hormonal treatments were successful; indeed, when he complained to his physician at Callen-Lorde about the slow pace of his change, she increased his medication doses. It was easy for me to support his request for vitamins and iron tablets and to follow his effort to "build muscles," as he put it, by attending a local gym, and to suggest, more than once, that he might someday no longer need Haldol to prevent relapse to depression. I also suggested he keep SSI informed of his earnings, lest they come back later to recoup their support payments. In a collegial way we discussed the clinical issues some of his clients presented.

By the time our work together ended he could see that the way forward was in his hands, and that the steps and timing were his to choose and carry out. He announced that if SSI imposed a limit on his savings, he would ask for full-time employment and forego support payments. As with most of his announcements, he did not act immediately, but he eventually did so, and more important, he knew that, somehow, he could. He found himself a nurse who had transferred from Pathways to Callen-Lorde, so that he was ultimately less dependent on my support. By accepting limited but symbolically important tasks his employment agency supervisor assigned him, the two of them developed a working relationship, marked by mildly teasing banter, which both tolerated. He was no longer the conflicted and uncertain adolescent he had been when we met.

Post-script

I had learned that Victor was one of the two former Pathways patients of mine who over the past year was receiving supported housing services from one of the Jamaica outreach teams of the Post-Graduate Center for Mental Health. The administration there put me in touch with the leader of that team. I was anticipating a favorable update on Victor's progress through the transition to masculine appearance and lifestyle. But I was in for a shocking disappointment. It was that he had recently relapsed to a level of symptoms more severe and disturbing to him than any I had encountered in our work together. I reported this unexpected downturn to the sexual disorders specialist at Columbia, whom I had consulted shortly after Victor's initial revelation of his transgender identity. This specialist commented on the rarity of the emergence of such symptoms, suggesting I might describe them to a group of his colleagues, but that has not yet been possible, because I have had no contact with Victor. In follow-up e-mails and calls the team leader reported that he had improved somewhat on medication and intended to call me, but that has not yet occurred. Therefore, I changed his first name and initial, to protect his anonymity.

Chapter 6
Richard G.

The trajectory of my work with Richard G. reveals itself in the pattern of my notes of our meetings. For the first 4 years one brief note a month was all it took; for the final nine months the rate doubled, and each note was much longer. The level of care needed to maintain him had increased significantly, but both phases reflect the same attributes of his character: kindness, loyalty, perseverance, and independence. Without these his story would have been merely sad, rather than uplifting and inspiring, and his decline would have been unmanageable in a community setting.

Personal and Psychiatric History

When I first met him, he was 55 and living alone, separated from his wife and long out of touch with his two adult children. His son was married and living in North Carolina, pursuing an Army career. His daughter lived in Delaware, and the relationship with her had once been "beautiful." Earlier in his life he had supported his family by working as a handyman, a burglar alarm technician, a carpet cleaner at the World Trade Center, and a shipping clerk, earning up to $500 a week. He had maintained contact with his mother, until her death six years earlier, and with a brother, whom he described as having been "a high-ranking police official," until his death, one and one-half years earlier. Since these losses he had felt, "I'm on my own." He heard rarely from a sister in The Bronx, and though he mentioned a girlfriend once, he had no regular contact with anyone outside our team. He explained that he preferred to spend most of his time in his apartment, listening to music on CD's, playing bass guitar, learning to paint, and cooking.

His father had served in the Air Force for 20 years before retiring. In adolescence Richard had gotten into trouble "for fighting," and was sent to Lincoln Hall [Boys' Haven], where the degree of structure, in contrast with what he called "my chaotic

© Springer International Publishing Switzerland 2016
W. Tucker, *Narratives of Recovery from Serious Mental Illness*,
DOI 10.1007/978-3-319-33727-2_6

family life," had apparently proven constructive. He described it fondly as a place "where we shoveled snow off the ice and played hockey on the pond." While there, he earned a GED. On release, at 18, had tried to enlist in the military, as his father had done, but was rejected for a health reason and given a 1-Y (deferred) classification.

That reason, most likely, was the paranoid schizophrenia from which he must already have been suffering as an adolescent, and which he presented to me as his diagnosis at our first meeting. He described his paranoia by explaining, "I'm watched so closely that I need protection. People don't treat me with respect, and male prostitutes call me names."

As is frequently the case with those carrying his diagnosis, his thinking was consistently clear and logical, and his thought pattern was never worse than slightly tangential, and his thought content, somewhat idiosyncratic—e.g., "I brush my teeth with Ajax and shampoo, because toothpaste makes me gag." His principal desire was to be left alone except for rare intrusions. As he put it, perhaps acknowledging some loneliness, "I have people to talk to, but I keep to myself." That preference was later to be tested severely by an incident involving apartment repair.

He had another problem, as well: he had abused street drugs for years, and though he had discontinued them some time before we met, on several occasions he remarked that "if I worked and had money now, I'd be right back on drugs, [because] they make me friendlier toward people," adding that, when he first came to Pathways, 5 years before me, he had "just gotten out of jail for crack." He explained that he had learned to avoid people in order to avoid more fighting, and street drugs, by avoiding people who used them. It is a measure of his self-awareness and self-control that he remained off street drugs without the help of a 12-step program. During the time of our meetings, he often used alcohol and occasionally showed up with it on his breath; nevertheless, I was never concerned that he had relapsed to drugs.

About a year into our meetings he developed an ingenious way to demonstrate both to himself and to us his determination to "stay clean": whenever he would meet with me or come to our office, he would bring me or another team member a bottle of orange or cranberry juice. As he explained, "When I stop bringing it, then you can worry." Several times he commented that, "not being on drugs, I've saved up more than you would believe." Indeed, the one occasion when he felt accused by team members of having relapsed and was refused access to some small savings he had put aside and described himself as having been "angry," it seemed to me that he was, rather, more hurt at being mistrusted.

His third and final problem was heavy smoking.

Engagement and Stability

Prescribing appropriate medication for him could not have been simpler. During our first four years, his dose of risperidone fluctuated between 4 and 8 mg daily, according to his requests, and his requests for Benadryl, a non-habit-forming sleep aid, were similarly reasonable. His view of their benefits would qualify easily as insight, to anyone who cared to score him on that item: "Medication helps me deal with loneliness and stress." He could even identify the source of his adherence: "My grandmother told me what to do and didn't have to tell me twice."

In return he asked for very little. His one room was furnished mostly with a couple of mattresses, along two walls, and perhaps a single chair. At any given time there were several CD players scattered about, never more than one of them functioning. The once-white walls of the kitchen alcove were spattered with yellow stains of cooking oil. Frying pans, some of them containing food residues, stood atop several of the burners. The room reeked of tobacco smoke.

Yet this was his world, where he spent most of his days, practicing his guitar and listening to recordings. Early on in my visits, I saw that his guitar strings were of rubber, and that they produced only the faintest sound. One day, walking to his neighborhood, I noticed some nylon ones in a shop window and during my next visit, offered to purchase them for him. He demurred but must have noted my offer, because he later replaced them on his own with steel ones, to my relief: a step up for him.

Besides showing up at my office monthly, he must have made periodic excursions to pick up food and other supplies, because toward the end I learned that, rare as these had been, he had managed to make a favorable impression on neighbors and even on casual strangers. They must have been impressed with his quiet dignity, just as we at Pathways regularly were.

One incident illustrates how limited his social interactions remained. His super suspected a gas leak in his apartment and had called the local fire department. Then he accompanied them on their visit, taking the opportunity to press me to transfer Richard elsewhere. He cited the casual housekeeping but more likely, I figured, was trying to forestall the landlord's responsibility to perform the required repainting. Richard remained cooperative and fairly calm throughout the whole incident, though he wondered whether the super "used a gas meter outside my door." He acknowledged the gas leak but attributed it to the extinction of a pilot light on the stove. It was clear that Richard had not contributed to the leak in any way. Once the stove was repaired, and the pilot light functioned again, the super seemed mollified, saying there was no longer any problem with his staying on. To forestall any future threats, I asked the super to call me if one ever arose again.

But the gas leak was not the major problem with the state of his apartment: water was. Over the course of the next 9 months Richard complained to the super about the impending collapse of his bathroom ceiling, due to water leaking from pipes in the floor above. A flimsy past effort at repair had already proven inadequate. Finally, the buckling and cracking became so threatening that he would no longer use the toilet. He feared being caught under falling plaster, so he took to using a bucket outside the bathroom door. I saw what he meant and could not fault him for what he did. The pressure on the super to act responsibly was mounting. But Richard had contributed his own share to the delays: because of his distrust of strangers, he had three times refused entry to the repairmen sent by the super. Now

Richard himself decided it was time to move to another apartment, and he offered me the customary soft drink to prove that his judgment was still intact.

During the wait for this move, which extended over another half-year, he and I focused mainly on his neglect of his general health. He seemed to be delaying seeking care for his hypertension. He excused his behavior with, "I'd need a courier to find a primary care doc, since the five I went to, weren't right. I'll go, but I'm in no rush: I'm trying to be good, drinking milk, eating cabbage, carrots, and ground beef." He avoided my recommendation that he visit the primary care doctor at the local Medicaid clinic, who was welcoming and attentive to several of our team's patients. When he finally managed to get a checkup at the Jamaica Hospital clinic, he reported being told he was in good health. That can hardly have been the case, and he was unable to give me the physician's name or bring me the results of his lab tests; however, I understood I was not to press him.

Finally, the new apartment came through, and though there was again a problem with the bathroom ceiling, this one had been satisfactorily repaired, "so," he concluded, "no problems!" He was pleased to have gotten a fresh start, where he could resume his playing guitar and listening to music, whenever he had a working CD player. As with Gary (Chap. 2), that remained a challenge. Fruit drinks were not his only gift to me: one Christmas he presented me with a pocket calculator and a small flashlight, and he brushed aside my attempt to refuse them by adding that he had "ten more." He continued to insist on chaining and padlocking his door, but he never failed to open it and welcome me or any of my team members.

I think you would have to agree that he was quite a gratifying patient. He maintained stability in the face of two potentially devastating psychiatric conditions, paranoid schizophrenia and polysubstance abuse. He expressed satisfaction with his lifestyle and incremental progress, however circumscribed and modest. And he asked so little of us in the way of helping him manage. I looked forward to our continuing monthly meetings.

So far, so good: all I needed to do was resist the temptation to ask him for more engagement, a request that would have been for my sake, not for his.

Systemic Health Issue

Then, after four years without missing a single meeting, he failed to show up. I set off for his new apartment, but I had mistakenly taken the address for the old one, so no one answered my knock. I returned the next day to the new address, but again, there was no answer, and this time, I was concerned: something was up, and my chart entry, a supposition that he was merely out on an errand, was just to cover myself.

When I returned the next week, the mystery was resolved, and both my confidence in him and my concern were confirmed. I learned that he had somehow managed the previous day to crawl across the floor and unlock his door to let in a team member, who found him lying on the floor of his apartment, emaciated and dehydrated. She had called 911 to have him rushed by ambulance to Jamaica Hospital. Now I hurried there to meet with the ER director and a neurosurgeon, who described to me the 4-cm metastasis they had discovered in his brain, and further, its presumptive origin, a carcinoma in his lung that was itself so large as to cause a shift in the symmetry of his lungs. They directed me to him, where he lay on a stretcher, barely able to speak, unable to direct the movements of his right arm or leg, and shaky. I recall that it was his shakiness and lack of coordination, rather than weakness, which struck me; later, the surgeon told me the metastasis was in his cerebellum, thus confirming my impression about the nature of his symptoms.

Richard requested and gulped down a cup of water, holding it in his left hand. The plan was to transfer him to Maimonides Hospital in Brooklyn for removal of the brain lesion and placement of a shunt from the blocked ventricles of his brain down into a vein in his neck, to relieve the intracranial pressure. For the first time I called his eldest sister, the family matriarch, in Atlanta, learning from her that, by a fortunate chance, she had just visited him the previous week after having lost touch with him for seven years prior to his arrival at Pathways.

A week later, on the postoperative recovery unit at Maimonides, he appeared miraculously improved. Though unable to raise himself up from his bed, he greeted me, shook my hand, and requested, this time from me, the customary bottle of orange juice: I certainly owed him a few of those! He denied pain or discomfort, managing to communicate, in spite of considerable difficulty in forming words, that he intended "to be okay, come home, and come to the clinic tomorrow." This sounded like both a wish and a promise, but it was to take quite a while longer than that.

I visited him next, a month later, at the nursing home to which he had been transferred for rehabilitation and for the duration of his radiation therapy treatments at a facility nearby, where he had already undergone a dozen of them. His sister had flown in from Atlanta and was in attendance. We were to begin eight months of communication about her brother's status by phone and, when she could, in person. Richard himself was up and walking, his coordination was restored, his speech was clear, and his entreaty to be allowed to return to his apartment as soon as possible was foremost in his mind.

My role in facilitating the process of meeting his request involved coordinating the necessary contacts with the radiation oncologist, who added a grim prognosis to his description of the treatments; with the primary care physician at the nursing home; and with the visiting nurse service, all of whose approvals were required for his discharge. As you may imagine, many questions were raised by all of them about the advisability of doing so, since it was clear to all of them, as well as to me and my team, that allowing him to try to manage at home was unsafe. But his sister was unwavering in her support of his preference, which he highlighted by refusing her offer to bring him home to Atlanta to live out the remainder of his life with her. Taking a page from her book, I plunged ahead. Still, it took another ten weeks to get him back to his apartment.

Restabilization and Death

I took a team member along for my first visit, both because I knew there would be a lot to do, and because I knew I would need the team's cooperation in order to carry out the ambitious attempt to maintain him as safely as possible at home. He appeared emaciated, short of breath, struggling to swallow and to speak, and unable to move about except with the use of a walker and wheelchair. Still, he assured us that, as usual, he was having no pain or discomfort and was "glad to be home." He asked that we not discard his filthy pillowcase and coverlet but agreed to let us have them washed.

It came as no surprise when the visiting nurses pulled out early, citing with some justification that he would not let unknown persons in, and that their agency could not guarantee scheduling consistency to those it assigned. Even their suggestion that he accept a live-in aide was, of course, doomed from the start, given his preference for privacy, and also given, as it turned out, his having too restrictive a form of Medicaid to cover that service. Even my emendation that the aide's visits could be restricted to a few times a week did not persuade him.

Though he deteriorated steadily over the next five months, reaching the end precisely at the time the radiation oncologist had predicted, his spirits never flagged, due only in part to our ability to respond to his modest requests. The larger part was surely due to his courage. That kind of courage, in the face of real danger, was familiar to me from the example of many people with schizophrenia I have known over many years (Section "How these Narratives Emerged").

Two team members alternated in their visits, and I increased the frequency of mine. His sister visited also, for several days, to assure herself that things were going as well as they might, given the circumstances. His coordination improved somewhat, allowing him to move about enough to get to the kitchen and to the bathroom, by walker and wheelchair. He began maintaining his new apartment somewhat more fastidiously than he had his original one, or, perhaps, it was simply that he went out less. In the beginning he managed to heat up some items, such as French fries from McDonald's, demonstrating for me how he could operate the gas stove, though in the end he acknowledged having been reduced to making sandwiches of luncheon meats, which I confirmed by checking out his refrigerator. As expected, the fruit juice regimen persisted, at least for a while.

We continued to negotiate around his insistence on a chained door, and he compromised by attaching it only to a hook, rather than to a padlock. When he requested a small TV to watch movies from his bed, and Pathways was unable to arrange a cable connection promptly, he settled for a small DVD player and a few disks. At first he was taking an antiemetic, an anticonvulsant, antibiotics for TB, vitamins to counteract the depletion caused by the antibiotics, and a reduced dose of my risperidone, but I was gradually able to eliminate all of these, one at a time, to simplify his regimen, without noticeable ill-effect.

The issue of cigarettes was another story. Though his partial SSI had been reduced to $30/month, he had managed to save up $115 in an account held at

Pathways, and he requested I use some of it to provide him with cigarettes. He insisted he needed them, "so I could talk better." Generally, I complied, but when he proposed spending $70 of what remained for them, I balked. In response to my best efforts he agreed to have me take only $30 and spend it on a box of cigars instead.

On his sister's next visit the three of us discussed his wishes for how we should respond, if his condition deteriorated further. He told us he preferred to have no more medical care, "unless I need it, in your opinion or in my sister's." Could we have hoped for a clearer response?

After two months at home he seemed no weaker than on his arrival there. He was no longer cooking, as noted above, but managed to subsist on fruit juices, ice cream, and chips. He was still navigating his apartment by walker and by wheelchair, thus getting himself to the toilet. One day he surprised me—shocked was more like it—by bringing himself from his apartment all the way to my office unassisted. If his goal was to persuade me to release all his unexpended funds, he succeeded.

A month later, I decided to take him on a shopping trip to local stores, in order to assess his coping skills, continued mobility, and judgment. I wheeled him out the door and helped him inside our van. Our first stop was for new batteries for his headset, and he duly doled out the funds for me to use. In the local supermarket he wanted to purchase hamburger, but when I reminded him there were a dozen frozen patties in his refrigerator already, he moved on. A community resident, recognizing him after a long absence, approached us and gave him a small amount of money, unsolicited. Another one, on our way out, commented to me, "He's such a fine man." He clearly needed more help getting back up into his seat in the van than previously, and I took the opportunity to ask again whether he would want me to hospitalize him if he were in immediate danger. Again, he said he would leave that up to me.

On our arrival back at his apartment I felt the need to recheck his orientation and was relieved when he was able to name the day and month correctly. That quick exam should not have been necessary: cerebellar problems do not cause loss of orientation. It must have been my need alone. He was now weakened to the point that, when asked to repeat something he had said too softly, the effort to comply exhausted him. Though he communicated that swallowing was becoming difficult, I was pleased to watch him put away one-half cup of ice cream, nevertheless.

Five months into his return home, I noted a row of Ensure bottles lined up on the floor at the head of his mattress, each one filled with urine. I asked the obvious question, but he insisted he was still able to get himself to the bathroom if he wanted to. His claim that he was still making himself sandwiches was belied by the unopened packages of meat and cheese in his refrigerator. I was beginning to concur with our team members, who visited several times a week, that he might soon need hospitalization on a medical unit, even as he entreated me, now in a whisper, to let him remain where he was.

A week later I visited him on a medical unit at Queens General Hospital, where he had been admitted because of dehydration. This had caused an elevation in his calcium level, which had made him sufficiently miserable that he had offered no objection to hospitalization; however, on receipt of intravenous fluids he seemed to be recovering once again. The unit physician was contemplating a discharge home, in accordance, as you have long since come to expect, with the patient's expressed wishes. But it was not to be: he died peacefully the next day, a few hours after a visit from one of his nephews. As his sister put it, "I guess God just called him home."

It was our practice at Pathways to arrange a small memorial service when one of our clients died. We were pleased that our patient advocate at the time, who had known Richard, at least in passing, was present to give his impression, as did several team members. Our nurse practitioner, Marcia Campbell, herself a Seventh Day Adventist and the most comfortable of all of us with spiritual matters, handled that part of the brief ceremony. Richard's sister, of course, attended, along with one of his grandnephews, and they expressed their appreciation for what we had done for him, as well as for the modest service. "I never knew my uncle," the young man told us, "until now, when I learned how other people saw him."

Post-script

Because of our many cordial contacts throughout the course of Richard's last illness I was not surprised by his sister's receptiveness and understanding, when I contacted her with my request that she provide consent, more than 5 years after our last communication. She asked that I send her a copy of my narrative by e-mail, and she carefully examined and approved it, with only a small number of factual corrections, which I have duly included. She expressed no concerns about her brother's anonymity. She added that my call had come just in time, because she was planning to move to another city, where it might have proven more difficult to locate her.

Chapter 7
Maria C.

Personal and Psychiatric History

From our first meeting Maria C. burst out of the starting gate and began a race to the finish, never to be distracted by looking right or left. She was a single, Latina mother in her early 30s. She had two daughters, nine and five. She had her own clear, reasonable idea of her diagnosis. She had not taken any medication for it, due at least in part to her not having consistently met with any Pathways psychiatrist, though she had concretely benefitted from other supportive services over the 7 years she had been a client there. Housing was surely the first of these. Prior to coming to Pathways she had been homeless and had temporarily lost her first child to agency care, due to accusations of prostitution (perhaps true) and substance abuse (almost certainly not true). Improved general health was a second one. Whereas she had required three trips to emergency rooms to manage her own asthma in the previous year, she was now managing it adequately at home—a fortunate development, because her younger daughter was beginning to suffer from it as well. A third was having sufficient time to attend to her daughters' considerable needs. Both were in special education classes, the older one already diagnosed with ADHD, and the younger one soon to join her.

From her description of her own symptoms as consisting principally of "problems focusing," it was not difficult to conclude that she suffered from the same condition, herself; indeed, on the occasion of our final meeting, five and one-half years later, when I described her to her new psychiatrist as suffering from ADD, she corrected me by reporting that, as a child, she had shown hyperactivity as well, and thus qualified for the full-blown ADHD picture.

© Springer International Publishing Switzerland 2016
W. Tucker, *Narratives of Recovery from Serious Mental Illness*,
DOI 10.1007/978-3-319-33727-2_7

Initial Treatment

A theme of our ensuing work together was to be her daughters' reenactments of many of her own difficult developmental experiences, and this theme was to be both a source of reassurance and hope, and also one of pain and concern. As she put it, much later on, summarizing so much of what they had shown, "they're just like me at their age, so I understand them, even before they tell me what's happened." This reenactment extended back into her own past, as well: one of the major areas in which her focusing was a problem was her housekeeping, which had been contaminated from early childhood by her mother's demands that she clean up her room, reinforced by repeatedly hitting her over the head with a spoon,. Thus, as an adult and mother, she often found herself avoiding the housekeeping altogether by going off to the local library "to surf the Internet."

She lost little time getting down to work. A month after our first meeting, she elaborated on her symptoms, adding that she had "trouble concentrating, was easily frustrated, and lost the focus of a conversation if it was not 'interesting.'" She requested stimulant medication for the specific purpose of being able to help her daughters with their homework, and she presented this request so readily, that I was puzzled she had gone so long without it. I may have asked a consultant in child psychiatry back my home base, Columbia, for a recommendation, and thus landed upon Concerta, described as a newer version of Ritalin (methylphenidate), with which I was more familiar, but even this substitution was to teach us both something, not too far down the line. A month later, she was reporting that, though she herself could recognize little change, others, including her sister, who helped often with household chores, and her older daughter, were already telling her that she was calmer and more focused, less "overly cheerful" and instead, "more mature," able to stay seated longer and, thereby, to hold longer conversations. She wrapped it up with words that any psychiatrist treating such patients is pleased to hear, because they reflect self-awareness: "I guess you have to be on the outside to see it."

As if that were not enough of an improvement, she also reported that, according to her primary care physician, her chronic iron-deficiency anemia, long attributed, rightly or wrongly, to having the recessive trait version of the hemophilia from which two of her brothers had suffered, and for which she had long been taking iron supplements, had somehow resolved itself. This dividend was surely only coincidental, but discovering it only resulted from her following through with an appointment with the hematologist she may otherwise not have managed to keep. We still had a long way to go together with much backing-and-filling, but her energy and determination had already shown the direction she was capable of taking, once she chose one for herself.

From then on, over the course of the next five years, she focused on several goals that will appear very much like those in the lives of people without mental illnesses: dealing with medication issues, maintaining her apartment, supporting and protecting her young girls, which included dealing with the Administration for Children's Services (ACS), the city's child protective agency, working at several successive jobs—some simultaneously, serving in the elected role of peer advocate, relating to a boyfriend, and moving on to a lesser level of support. Even though, of course, these were all interwoven temporally, each of them deserves its own mini-narrative, so that is how I will present them.

Progress Toward Longer-Term Goals

The first one concerned her medication. Many people find stimulant medication helpful for brief or extended periods in their lives, to accomplish specific or longer-term goals. A few of my private patients have used it in order to be able to complete books they have struggled to write; others, to maintain adequate functioning at work. Thus, the attentional problem Maria was having would not, by itself, have qualified her as having serious mental illness; rather, it was only the last straw which, added to the burden of her early traumatic experiences and of unsupported motherhood, had driven her into the streets.

Her issues with stimulant medication were rather straightforward. As just noted, she found it immediately effective in the view of others close to her. Her one complaint was that it caused her to become "too emotional," frequently to the point of tears, and therefore, she was reluctant to take it regularly. As soon as she began working, however, she found it indispensable; thereafter, the only reason she occasionally skipped doses seemed to be the primary reason for taking it in the first place and for causing her frequently to be late in refilling her prescriptions, namely, distractibility. On the other hand, this very lateness demonstrated that she was clearly not abusing it—not that she needed to prove it. An interesting complication arose, a few years into this pattern, when she was forced to switch to the older drug, Ritalin (=methylphenidate), by a new Medicaid policy stipulating that she would have had to come up with a $3 co-pay to continue with Concerta, unless the older drug had proven problematic for her. As it happened, she found Ritalin to be free of the side effect of overemotionality and preferred it to Concerta, though she continued to miss doses, just as before.

The second one concerned her homemaking. Her issues with maintaining her apartment were anything but straightforward. The Sisyphean task any single parent faces in keeping things in order while trying to raise latency-aged children was complicated, for her, both by her early associations to housekeeping, and by her desire for time to devote to her own personal development in the larger world, which drove her out of her apartment whenever she could find a reason to go. On special occasions, such as preparing for visits from ACS or showing the apartment off to me, she would make a special effort, but her heart was not in it. Two episodes will highlight the problem. The first coincided with the summer day after a party she had thrown to attract potential Avon customers. She had done her best to put the apartment back in order, but I noticed some huge garbage bags in her kitchen. Opening one of them up, I saw a horrific sight: the leftover food was infested with thousands of crawling, white maggots. Then I noticed that her windows had no screens, and she acknowledged it was hard to keep the flies out. It took me till the next summer, and the occasion of yet another visit from ACS scheduled for the next day, to take the obvious step: I went down to the local Home Depot and bought her a set of adjustable window screens. These solved the problem for good.

The second episode involved me only indirectly. I had heard from our team that her apartment had been infested with bedbugs, and that I should be careful about sitting down on any covered chair during a home visit. The apartment seemed clean enough, but I maintained my skittishness and sat only on wooden chairs. Later, I learned Lascelles Black, our agency's family therapy supervisor, who had also been crucial to Gary's therapy and to Victor's, brought home the bedbugs from her apartment, and he had had to dispose of much of his furniture to get rid of them. Pathways replaced Maria's furniture—but not his.

In the struggle to support and protect her young girls the theme is again about feeling overwhelmed and needing help, but in a different way, namely, about keeping others from interfering with her parenting. It was never clear to me how ACS got involved in the first place, but for two and one-half years that agency presented the constant threat, in her mind, at least, of taking them away from her. She had several theories about who initially reported her to that agency. One was that a neighbor, whom she had regularly paid to supervise them, was angry at having been dismissed, and made the call in retaliation, accusing her of neglect. Another was that her children's step-grandfather—i.e., the husband of her children's father's mother, was the one. She suspected that his interest in her elder daughter, who had turned ten, was an illicit one, and her suspicion, unfortunately, was supported by her several accounts by the child of being placed in his lap and invited to "drive" (her daughter's word) his car, and of her coming home regularly from these visits agitated and "rebellious," often starting fights with her younger sister.

Nor were Maria's fears hypothetical: she had been sexually abused as a child, herself. You might ask why she permitted the visits to continue at all, but such a question would only show a failure of understanding of the real pressures a parent under ACS's watch is subjected to: the grandfather regularly threatened that if she interfered, he would report her to ACS for poor parenting. Gradually, though, whatever the source of ACS's concerns, they came to take Maria's side. Once she provided them with the requested reports from the psychiatrists who prescribed her girls their stimulant medication, and who attested to her faithfulness in keeping most of the scheduled visits, the agency relented and closed her case. Perhaps they had become aware and were impressed, as I certainly was, that both girls had gradually begun doing better in school. She even managed to convince a teacher to prevent the older daughter from cutting class, which a boy in her class was urging on her.

The third one concerned her several jobs. Maria was hard at work as a teacher's assistant—"tutor to toddlers," she called it—within 6 months of our first meeting, and the job lasted nine months, making it the longest she had held a position up to that point in her life. Over the next five years, she was only rarely and briefly unemployed. The stimulant medication may have played a role in enhancing her self-confidence, insofar as she announced more regular adherence once she began working, but the larger factor must have been her own determination.

Supplementing her meager SSI allotment was only a secondary objective: the primary one was to express herself through the work, to personalize it. Indeed, two of her employers were stretched as thin as she was, but she refused to give up before they did. One was a woman whose business was to operate a small day care group, which lasted until several of the financially strapped parents failed to pay for her services. The other was the owner of a store selling religious articles, continually in financial straits, where Maria eventually began bringing in various stimulating perfumes she had acquired and offering spiritual counseling along with the objects themselves. The high point of her work-life was her involvement, off-and-on, with Avon, the pretext for the party mentioned above. When it appeared that she was spending more to buy their products than she earned in commissions by selling them, she acknowledged needing to take a second look. That led to her paying for a trip to North Carolina to attend a Market America meeting, to learn more about how businesses operate; however, the cost of that trip itself became an added financial burden. Even when she realized she was losing money, she asserted Avon would "teach [her] cosmetology," which was her objective. She had spent $135 on a camera to start a modeling portfolio, "money I could have used for other things."

The high point of her upward trajectory was her turning up at our office one day, dressed in a slinky, full-length, blue-sequined dress, which she had worn to a fashion show the previous weekend. She announced that, "I thought that would never happen, because I have a burn scar down my left leg from my waist to my ankle. Being there made me feel like a million bucks." She looked like it, too.

The fourth goal was a continuation of the previous one. Two years into our work together, she successfully campaigned for the position of Peer Advocate by her fellow Pathways clients. This role was what the title implied, i.e., interceding with our staff on behalf of fellow clients unable to advocate adequately for themselves. She began, earnestly enough, doing just that. Calculating that it took up 13 h of her time each month, she set up a routine of office hours in which she was available to hear about problems and complaints. Within a few months she reported, "This 'consumer business' is hard: you can't please everyone, but it hurts not to—for example, I wish [another client] had told me earlier about the threat of having ACS take her baby away." Apparently she fulfilled her fellow clients' expectations, because, a year later, she was reelected to the position, much to her satisfaction. In her second year she hit upon an original and highly successful twist: holding monthly meetings at which several fellow clients at a time could gather to discuss one another's issues. "Many of them won't talk one-on-one, but they will in a group." Though she realized this position took further time away from her girls, she was exultant, announcing, "Finally, I've found something I like!"

The fifth was barely a distraction. Her two years in this position immediately followed upon an incident that would likely have distracted someone less determined, but it preoccupied me much more than it did her. One afternoon, in front of her apartment, she was caught in a cross-fire between unknown assailants and was shot in her left thigh. She had gone to a local ER and been treated and released. Other than reporting she had pain in most positions, especially at night, and showing me the wound, she seemed rather unconcerned. I worried about the possibility of lead poisoning, given that the bullet was still in place, and about damage to local tissue. I called the ER and scheduled a follow-up appointment with a surgeon. She and the surgeon continued to be unconcerned, and they turned out to be correct in their more measured assessment of the wound. Over the course of two months, the bullet gradually worked its way to the surface and caused no further problems other than a few extrusions of bloody fluid.

The sixth involved an intimate relationship. Coincident with the beginning of her role as Peer Advocate, she began a relationship with a new boyfriend—the first one I heard about. Within a few months she was "considering all options," which included both moving immediately with him to Puerto Rico, and on the other hand, taking things slowly, "just trying to enjoy the moment." How invested she was in this relationship was never clear to me. She described him as "unreliable" at times, but she was also aware that her girls were very fond of him; indeed, they feared more than she did that the relationship would not last. Things continued in this way for two and one-half years. When she had to make a brief trip to Puerto Rico to visit her ill grandfather, she left the girls with this boyfriend and was delighted on her return to find that they had cleaned the apartment together. As she put it, "he gets along with them so well, it's 'crazy'!" But she also complained about his jealous tirades, telling him she was "not that kind of woman," and wondering to herself whether he were not doing something improper, himself, to make him suspect her. It was not long thereafter that they broke up, occasioning a meeting with Black, where he offered consolation for her double loss, both of the boyfriend, and, at the same time, of her best friend, a woman, due to illness, whom she mourned more. He added that her ability to grieve properly was itself a demonstration of the power of her stimulant medication, which permitted her to focus on an emotion long enough to understand it.

Step-Down to a Lesser Level of Services

The last in this listing of chapters of Maria's accomplishments was a successful graduation from ACT services, a newly introduced policy at Pathways for which Maria was an ideal candidate, as you will either have suspected from my account already or will readily imagine now. Fortunately for us both, this policy was so new that we were allowed to proceed, unharried, at our own pace—or rather, at hers, with me tagging along. The first step was for her to consolidate her gains. She was holding down two jobs, one in the religious articles store and another as a sales-person on a commission basis for Avon, as a result of which she was "almost up to date" in paying off her debts. Still, she was in no hurry to move on. Her first response to the idea was, "I feel good here and loved; it's safer having someone to see frequently; I've tried giving it [i.e., this level of support] up before, and it didn't work."

I must concede that I was not keen on this new policy, hopefully only out of belief in the maxim that dictates, "If it's not broken, don't fix it," rather than out of resistance to change; either way, I did not push the issue. A year later, however, she acknowledged being "willing to talk about it, but not yet ready to move on" to a supported housing program without ACT services. Through no fault of hers, the store could no longer employ her full-time. She took up with a new boyfriend—this time, one with a good job; still, some of you would say, wisely, she decided to "take it slowly." As in so many past situations, she relied on her sister to pick up her older girl after school and was comforted—somewhat—to learn that the daughter was angry at the boys who continued to pursue her. In the wake of these developments she reiterated that she "like[d] being seen six times a month: it makes me feel someone cares." She acknowledged being ready to move on from our program but expressed the wish at least to continue meeting both with Black and with me.

Further milestones passed: her older girl graduated from the eighth grade, and her younger one improved sufficiently in special education classes to be considered for mainstreaming. She gave me a tour of her clean apartment, to show me how much things had improved since our last one, three years before.

As the day of "graduation" neared, she asked for assistance in finding a new psychiatrist, suggesting the psychiatric clinic at Jamaica Hospital. She had felt a connection there, ever since receiving prenatal care for her first child, and the long-time receptionist there remembered her; still, she got no response to her application for services. Now the ball was clearly in my court. Two years after our first discussion of graduation, I accompanied her to the clinic to meet with her newly assigned psychiatrist. This woman was skeptical and even somewhat suspicious of why I was handing Maria off, not having been informed about the new, state-driven policy encouraging such a step-down. Had Maria ever been suicidal? What problems was she having with her stimulant medication? To cover all bases, she asked that I send a complete psychiatric and medical history—not an unreasonable request, but hardly the rule at the time. In return she announced that she would meet with Maria monthly and would arrange for a therapist to see her at least every 2 weeks. Maria hardly had a chance to speak at all during these formalities, and though I did not realize it at the moment, this was to be the last time I saw her. She was focused on the future and had no time for good-byes. I was the one feeling left behind.

Post-script

I expected Maria to continue to do well, and my expectation was confirmed. Having accompanied her to the clinic, as just noted above, I hoped to be able to contact her through her current psychiatrist or psychotherapist there. I was aware that proper protocol precluded my access to her current contact information, which, indeed, I did not seek. However, her therapist suggested I call during the time of her next scheduled visit, during which she asked Maria if she remembered me. The mention of Pathways jogged her memory, and we spoke briefly for the first time in 5 years, arranging to meet her at that clinic prior to her next appointment. She showed up on time, beaming, as usual, and reported that she was, as before, working multiple jobs. Currently these included as an independent travel agent, a chocolate seller, and an Avon salesperson. Her elder daughter, now 19, divided her time between Maria and her father's family, apparently without ill effects. Her younger one, 15, was taking both mainstream and special education classes. She asked me to read aloud my description of our encounters. Then she responded that I could publish them, using her name.

Chapter 8
Alex A.

This story concerns a young man who should never have been relegated to the mental health system in the first place. He got there, nevertheless, because that system is the default option for scooping up anyone who shows disordered behavior, even as an adolescent, and because no one in a position of authority in that system identified the obvious source of his disordered behavior in time to redirect him out of that system promptly and into the appropriate one.

Issues in Childhood and Adolescence

From the time he was a toddler his mother recognized that there was something different about him. "He always played alone, not with other kids—he wasn't like my daughter (his older sister)." Consequently, she took him at the age of 3 ¾ years to the Jamaica Health Station, from which he was referred to Queens' Advanced Center for Psychotherapy. There they had the good fortune to fall upon a psychologist who provided weekly behavioral treatment sessions for the next 6 years. As a result of these, Alex A. progressed from a vocabulary of 10 words in English and 20 in Spanish to nearly age-appropriate language skills, and even from special schooling to mainstreaming. Intelligence testing (WISC) at 9 would show a verbal IQ of 90 and performance IQ of 80, both within the normal range, but also "a significant weakness in social judgment." The benefits of his mother's efforts persisted for the next 6 years, so that, when he reached adolescence, he was able to matriculate at the John Adams High School.

Then, at 15, problems stemming from his underlying condition reemerged. In the absence of any specific event other than the march of puberty, he began to say that he was "depressed" and to show aggression toward his mother and older sister, punching them and pulling their hair. The pattern of this behavior was not clear to me, until we had worked together for several months, and I had received many reports from his family and from my team. He so easily felt provoked and so

© Springer International Publishing Switzerland 2016
W. Tucker, *Narratives of Recovery from Serious Mental Illness*,
DOI 10.1007/978-3-319-33727-2_8

frequently responded with sudden outbursts that seemed to be coming from nowhere, that it came as no surprise to learn that he had been referred repeatedly to the mental health system, even though he regularly settled down after only a few moments, regardless of any intervention or of none at all. He spent his next 7 years institutionalized, mostly in a state psychiatric hospital. From there he was discharged to a university hospital under the Second Chance program and from there to Pathways. There is a big problem with trying to access New York's developmental disability system, then called the Office of Mental Retardation and Developmental Disabilities (OMRDD), from within the mental health system. It requires a major shift in direction, and as a precondition of that shift, proof that the diagnosis of developmental disability was established before age 22. I had been around the public sector long enough to learn that assembling sufficient proof would be neither quick nor easy, even though, in Alex's case, there was plenty of it available.

Early on in our encounters I had a hunch that such behavior was due to a developmental disability rather than to a psychiatric disorder. Much later, once I got access to the initial evaluations, I would find that they provided specific, telling details: that he had been unable to name body parts except by echolalia [=imitation of the sound of the word], was unable to follow a two-step command (such as, "take off your coat and then sit down"), did not speak while playing, communicated mainly by gesture, scored well below age level on all intelligence tests except geometric shapes, and overall, related better to the test materials than to the examiner, who was therefore unable to distinguish noncomprehension from refusal. But these details were tucked away, and no one was looking for them yet.

It was not difficult to understand why psychiatrists treating him on inpatient units, whose first priority was to stabilize patients sufficiently for discharge, had neither the time nor the inclination to pursue getting hold of those evaluations. The crucial testing and behavioral observations dated from much earlier, and locating those early records is both highly time-consuming and outside the routine protocols of such units. For various systemic reasons which will become clearer shortly, it took me 2 years to get them, and even when I did, it took me several months more to get him access to OMRDD services.

For him, for his family, and for the ever-available but under-equipped mental health system, these delays had not been benign. Alex came to us only during the last half of my tenure at Pathways, and over the 2.5 years that we worked together, he required the services of 7 different community hospitals from Far Rockaway, in Queens, to Westchester County, in which he spent a total of ten months as an inpatient; 6 different community living arrangements; a major university medical center's special assessment system; and the enduring efforts of his indomitable mother and older sister, who, through a period of almost continuous abuse by him and worry about him, understood the goal and stayed the course. The eventually successful outcome of the change in treatment venue had positive significance for Alex's potential for change in the future, and at some level he was aware of that goal and endorsed it; he even shared our frustration that it was taking so long. Along the way it required more frequent encounters from me than for any other patient I worked with in my 6 years with this program—two and one-half per month, so that I saw him as frequently in our 2 ½ years as I did most of my patients in 6. As you may imagine, this kind of flexibility in my scheduling was an essential element in our agency's rulebook, one that encouraged clinicians to come up with the creativity that promoting recovery frequently requires.

Initial Treatment

When I first met Alex, I found him a pleasant, neat, somewhat chubby young man who looked and acted younger than his 22 years. His default presentation was one of friendly cheerfulness, and he was willing to play my game by trying to respond to the questions I posed, though his mind was elsewhere. He was caught up in the world of superheroes and action figures, rather than with the developmental and clinical issues I was supposed to pursue. He was vaguely aware of the events taking place around him and of other people's expectations but was almost completely unable to take them into account. Rather, he was preoccupied with what he took to be his problem in the first place, namely, that the proximity of other people, whether family or strangers, caused him pain. He knew they expected something from him, but their signals, sooner or later, inevitably seemed to him so contradictory. Considered in this way his confusion was heart-breaking, though up close, it did not feel so benign. It may help to illustrate the fantasy life he presented to tell you that his story begins with his reference to the horror film, "My Bloody Valentine" and ends with his reference to a similar film, "Halloween."

At the university psychiatric hospital unit where he had spent ten months prior to coming to our program, he had endorsed racing thoughts, panic attacks, crying spells, poor concentration, obsessions, and thoughts of jumping off a building "for no reason"—that is, he was never suicidal. In what must have been interpreted as a hallucination, he also reported "small slivers" of reality that flashed before his eyes, usually toward evening. On the basis of these symptoms he was diagnosed with schizoaffective disorder, a variety of schizophrenia, and prescribed whopping doses of clozapine for his hallucination, valproate for his mood swings, and venlafaxine for his obsessions. I noted at our first meeting that his ability to abstract appeared intact, which was for me—and would have been, for the old-timers among you—a tip-off that schizophrenia was unlikely, but I did not initially question the diagnosis in his record. He had passed some parts but not others required for his general education diploma (GED), though it was hard to attribute that failure to his condition alone, given that he had had no schooling past the middle of his sophomore year of high school.

He had been around more than a few psychiatrists before me, so he had learned to begin by asking for help with two problems related to his medication, first, that they made him drowsy all the time, and second, that they were not helping at all with his obsessions. I plunged ahead with efforts to fix both of these, the first, appropriately, but the second, not so, because I did not initially recall that obsessions are almost invariably part of his underlying condition. He also asked for help in preparing to retake his GED and, in the meantime, to join our program's weekly photography group, run by our art therapist, Rachel Romero, noting it was a hobby enjoyed by his sister and grandfather, two characters who are to appear several times in this story. He said he spent most of his time playing video games, which reflected the content of his fantasy life again and again. Later on he asked me who my favorite action figure was. When I told him it was Superman, he dismissed my choice as being "the ultimate boy-scout"—*touche!*—and asserted that his was Spiderman. This topic was also to return later as a suggestion for a potential career for him. Here, early on, it provided a source of pleasure, when he related how he had accompanied his sister, a New York policewoman, and her friends to a showing of "My Bloody Valentine" on her birthday. Otherwise, he never socialized outside his family.

Four months into our work, things were going along fairly smoothly. He said he liked having his own apartment and tried to keep it neat, something he learned how to do from "[his] mother's nurturing for many years." He said he "wasn't depressed anymore." In the month of his joining our program he had spent the Thanksgiving holiday with his family for the first time in 4 years. I had managed to cut both his clozapine and valproate in half without the emergence of noticeable problems, and he reported being less drowsy during the day. He was on good terms with our art therapist about what he called his "psychological pain," brought on by memories of physical abuse at the hands of his biological father. His parents were divorced when he was three, and they had had little actual communication thereafter.

His mother provided vivid accounts of just how aggressive he had been on numerous occasions. He had once pushed his younger half-sister down the stairs, so his mother was reluctant to have him live with them. She also reported he had been self-destructive, once jumping off the roof of a four-storey building—fortunately, without injury—and several times cutting himself, which she tried to prevent by putting all the kitchen knives away. Alex insisted he had only cut himself once but confirmed having brutally attacked his mother several times, pummeling and shoving her. She reported that he had had some temporarily satisfactory interactions with a male cousin, but that he had ultimately behaved badly, causing his cousin to break off the relationship. This may have been the precipitant of the jumping episode.

First Attempt at Redirecting Treatment

A note to myself at this time suggests that I was finally thinking about how to pursue my hunch that his diagnosis was Asperger's Disorder. When I told Alex, he recalled that a neurologist at the university hospital where he had spent time immediately before joining our program had raised a similar question. Still, I knew I was going to need a lot of expert support to prove that it was more than a hunch. The first step was to have him evaluated by someone with special expertise, whose judgment would carry weight with OMRDD. Fortunately, I knew Agnes Whitaker, the developmental psychiatrist Columbia Medical Center, where I was a faculty member; even more fortunately, she consented to provide the evaluation. Only later was I to learn that, because Medicaid itself did not cover such an evaluation, she had needed to dip into a special research account to pay for it, which she did, as a favor to me.

At his first visit she tested him extensively enough to be able to confirm my diagnosis. She explained to me that verbal strength in the face of mathematical deficiency is common in this condition and reminded me that obsessional symptoms are, too. While taking all of this in, Alex's mother, who had brought him there, revealed to us that she had just been told of a new threat, namely, that she might have breast cancer. She was much relieved to have at last found someone who understood him, because she feared that, if something happened to her, "No one [would] be left to care for him." This testing session turned out to be only the first of several.

Complications

Alex was willing to continue with whatever testing was necessary, but every day was a new struggle for him, and he was becoming impatient. "I've been acting irresponsible for the past two months, staying up all night, watching TV, talking back to everyone. I tell myself I'll never achieve happiness. I don't value life, because life isn't fair. I'm not clinically depressed or suicidal, but I'd like the pain to end. Last month I got pissed off at my stepfather for telling me to clean up my apartment, and another time, when I slammed the door in my mother's face, he asked me to apologize, but I just walked off."

Things escalated in a hurry. One day his sister called to tell me he had just smashed his eyeglasses and cell-phone, along with some furniture. She had taken him into her own apartment briefly, but he needed to be sent back to the university hospital from which he had come to our program 21 months before. There the psychiatrist accepted his new diagnosis but wanted to retain him anyway, believing, I supposed, that a holding action was all she had to offer. It took about an hour for me to drive there from Queens, but the ensuing visits were worth the effort. He spoke of being "in love" with his cousin's girlfriend, whatever that may have meant to him, many years after last having been in touch with him. His sister affirmed for me that this feeling was his way of remembering the good days of their earlier relationship. I was aware that aggressive outbursts were secondary consequences of his Asperger's Disorder, reflecting his exasperation over not being able to identify and express his feelings more clearly. So, I asked Alex if he thought he was ever able to contain his aggression toward his family. He replied, "I don't know any more. These days I try hard to think, but it doesn't work, so I do only a little of it." This wording is quite revealing of the precise nature of his disorder. His thinking was quite clear; furthermore, it would be hard for me to imagine how anyone could make up that reply.

Progress

Once he was released from the hospital, I took the next step, calling the OMRDD information service. I was told we would need a psychological report containing the results of his adaptive skills testing, which was already available from Whitaker's office, and of cognitive testing, which was still to be performed, along with my pulling together a psychosocial summary, a physical exam, a signed authorization to release his school records, and a description of his symptoms of Asperger's. On the positive side I was reassured that such a group home as we were seeking was indeed available, if he qualified for it.

To his sister I recommended Temple Grandin's book on living with Asperger's, asking her to share it with her mother for encouragement. I asked her also to help us get Alex's school and psychological treatment records and to take him along with her as proof of his approval for their release. She was unable to initiate the process herself, and in the end it was quite a surprise how we finally succeeded. At least I warned her that his problematic behavior was likely to continue in the meantime.

More Complications

Sure enough, Alex soon got himself hospitalized again, this time by running naked through a parking lot, something he had first done at 17 and several times thereafter. It took us several weeks to locate him, because he had chosen not to reveal his involvement with our agency and, further, to give his grandfather's name instead of his own. Thus, it took all the sleuthing skills of an astute social worker at Brooklyn's Woodhull Hospital, to which the police had taken him, to track us down, which she did by pursuing his mention of treatment by an ACT team in Jamaica, Queens. It was on one of my visits there that Alex and I discussed our respective favorite superheroes.

After a month he was released, only to disappear once again. This time we were unable to locate him for 2 months, despite the efforts of NYPD's Missing Persons Bureau, two Legal Aid attorneys, and his mother's sister, acting as the family's point person, all working together, though not always harmoniously. After all our leads had proven false, I received a chance phone call one day from a medical student training in psychiatry at Lincoln Hospital in The Bronx, who took the initiative to contact me. When I arrived there, Alex greeted me with the words, "You've finally come to see me." Barely containing my exasperation, I asked him why he had requested his family not be contacted. He responded that he was "annoyed" with them for no longer caring about him—an assertion that had been particularly hurtful to his sister, whom he refused to see when she later did try to visit him. The psychiatrist said he was ready for discharge but had failed three placement interviews at supervised residences. I was never certain whether all this behavior was a game or a manipulation, or whether Alex could tell the difference.

More Progress

Lincoln Hospital had advanced our case far beyond the mere holding action that the others had provided. The unit social worker on her own initiative applied for his school records from the Board of Education and had them sent to me; these were to prove dispositive in convincing OMRDD. Furthermore, the unit psychologist administered the MMPI, a psychological screening exam, which indicated the absence of any psychosis—a result confirming my initial impression and supporting the efforts underway to move him from ineffective psychiatric interventions to potentially effective ones available in the disability system.

Still More Complications and More Progress

All that remained now by way of gathering materials for our application was the cognitive testing back at Whitaker's evaluation center at Columbia. After his release from the hospital Alex cycled back to his room at the local YMCA, from which he was soon expelled for breaking a food warmer; to his uncle's house, which he was asked to leave after threatening the uncle's young children; to a psychiatric unit at Jamaica Hospital, where he presented himself after leaving his uncle's; and to a similar unit at Queens General, where he was committed after assaulting a retarded young man in the emergency room, after being rejected for the voluntary admission he had requested. His discharge needed to be timed precisely for the day of the scheduled cognitive testing. We planned to whisk him out one door and in through the next, a borough away. To set this course in motion, the unit psychiatrist needed approval from the departmental chief psychiatrist; again, cooperation was forthcoming.

The picture by now was becoming clear to everyone. Accompanied by his sister, Alex joined me at the appointed hour, and we drove together from Queens to upper Manhattan, a path by now more than familiar to us. Whitaker's research team psychologist confirmed that his IQ remained in the normal range and provided the suggestion that, under ideal circumstances, he might someday become engaged in helping create action-hero stories as a meaningful career. This might have been overly optimistic, but it also might not: Alex had done very well for 6 years with a behaviorally oriented treatment during his childhood; therefore, why should he not be able to benefit from such an approach as a young adult? I preferred to give both him and OMRDD the benefit of the doubt.

A month later, I got a call from a psychiatric resident at the sixth community hospital (out of seven), located in Far Rockaway, not far from an "A" train stop. The features were unchanged: he was found naked in a park, used his grandfather's name, assaulted a fellow patient by breaking his glasses, and threatened a staff member for requesting he change a TV channel. I took the first of these, his disrobing, as a childlike way of expressing a call for help, rather than as a psychotic symptom. The unit psychiatrist concurred with my diagnosis and later called me to offer Alex an unquestioned admission any time he needed it. Not only was this a gesture of good will, but it was also an affirmation of the kind of positive response Alex was capable of eliciting.

During that same visit, Alex and I traded action-figure stories again, but this time with a telling and unexpected twist: when I confused his reference to the Poke Man action-hero with the old Pokemon figure in a much earlier video game, he became visibly upset and frustrated, but instead of hitting out at me, he slapped his own wrist, hard. I suppose his reaction here will confirm what many of you think already, namely, that he had control over some of his aggressive outbursts and was selective in his responses; if so, you will concur with his stepfather, who believed Alex was harsher with those he took to be more tolerant of them. But I am not so sure: while it is true that he always spared our art therapist, Romero, and me, it is also true that he never injured anyone—neither staff nor family nor even strangers—so badly as to require medical treatment; indeed, after one such incident, the staff member he had assaulted came to our agency office to inquire whether she had done anything to provoke it. Thus, my guess would be that he was always exercising some measure of control, but that to read his aggression as instrumental would be only partly true. As he said so many times and in so many ways, "I want to be with people but not hang out with them." Who but someone with his condition could even imagine that?

After the Far Rockaway hospital experience, we moved him into one of the houses our agency owned. There were already three other residents there, Gary (Chap. 2), Seth (Chap. 9), and a third man. Each had his own room, so interaction with the others was as limited as each one chose. I suggested to Alex that he spend his days at a local library, reading about the action figures he fantasized about, and he took me up on it, reporting with delight that it was only a 10-min walk from the house. Nevertheless, he only lasted there a month before getting himself readmitted to the nearest community hospital, where he was already known. I had some pains to convince the unit psychiatrist not to petition to have him transferred to a state psychiatric hospital, which would almost surely have derailed for the foreseeable future our chances of proving his eligibility for developmental disability services. The psychiatrist went along, discharging him back to the house, while we all awaited the crucial meeting with OMRDD, set for the last day of 2010, now 2 ¼ years since he had come to our agency. Our contact there, the Associate Director for Queens, turned out to be the sort of public official one hopes to encounter, especially in difficult situations: informative, constructive, responsive, competent, reliable, and prompt; had he not been all of these, all our efforts would have dissipated, as we were all, by this time, close to exhausting our options—except Alex, of course.

The first reply we received was that the question of eligibility would have to be bumped up to OMRDD's Eligibility Committee, in view of Alex's extensive psychiatric history. That would take another month, because they met only in the first week of each month and needed a week to review the records, so we were put off till February. That was enough of a setback to send Alex back into the seventh and last community hospital, this one a different university hospital in Westchester

County, for breaking the bathroom mirror of a church. Soon discharged back to the house for the third time, he requested bed linens, which turned out to be a sign that he had decided to settle in, at least temporarily. This time, he remained there for 5 weeks, the longest period on his own and away from his family without a hospitalization since he had joined us.

Success

Then we got the long-awaited good news that he had been found eligible, and that he needed only to accept a three-month application period, an overnight stay in the residence, and an invitation to dinner. The family was asked to designate a social service agency to provide a case worker who, in turn, would make the formal application. That done, we were asked to gather together the letter of support from the OMRDD Associate Director for Queens; the psychological test results prepared by Whitaker's research team psychologist; the physical exam and psychosocial summaries provided by our program; and my attestation that he was a high-functioning autism patient, who would not need psychiatric treatment other than medication for sleep and for his thyroid, because he did not have a psychiatric disorder. I had no hesitation at all in providing such an attestation, but I can imagine the skepticism reflected in some of your faces, if you have read this far. But Asperger's Disorder, even though it was listed in the DSM-IV, was not a "psychiatric disorder," referable to the mental health system, as far as OMRDD was concerned; rather, it was their bread and butter.

At our final meeting Alex asked, "Now that we're so close to our goal, I can say that I feel very bad, but that isn't enough: am I evil, like the person in 'Halloween?'" I asked whether he could distinguish fantasy from reality, and he replied that he knew the film was fantasy, and that he had no desire to hurt anyone, but that he still had trouble dealing with the "rage that boils up inside [him]." That was good enough for me. What was good enough for him was hope, in particular, that the future might be better than the present or past.

Post-script

I had spoken in person and by telephone many times to Alex's older sister, an NYPD officer. I assumed that her consent was the appropriate one, given his diagnosis, even though he had never formally been deemed incompetent to consent to other aspects of his treatment. Fortunately for me, she had retained the same cell-phone number as before. In the interim she had been promoted to sergeant. In response to my offer to provide her with a copy of my narrative of her brother and their family's concerted efforts at getting him proper services, she replied cordially that she preferred to endorse what I had written, sight unseen, requesting only that I provide her with a copy of the book, once it appears. Thereupon, she called her brother, who provided me with the address of his current group home and echoed his sister's request for the finished product. He sounded cheerful and pleased with his current setting. As to his history of stability over the past 5 years and to his treatment, I neglected to obtain further information during that call. At my request his sister asked him to call me again, and he did so, but I never managed to reach him.

Chapter 9
Seth S.

Initial Meeting

Seth did not so much introduce himself to me as descend upon me. He showed up at my office door for our first meeting, toting a moderate-sized duffel bag, from which he proceeded to unpack an array of personal items: T-shirts, sweatshirts, basketball shorts, a leather motorcycle jacket, and a crash helmet—all obtained, he assured me, at bargain prices. After showing me each one, he awaited my admiring response, before repacking it into the duffel bag. Then he handed me plastic bags containing several large manila envelopes, stuffed with clippings from national newspapers, and many free, local newspapers in their entirety, along with advertising fliers and brochures, marked up to highlight articles of particular relevance. These he introduced for me to peruse at my leisure. He also produced tickets and ticket stubs from rock concerts and other types of contemporary pop music I was less familiar with, as well as from a range of professional sporting events—some past, some future—and fliers from self-help meetings and public policy events he had attended, to show how he kept himself occupied. Once displayed, these followed the items of clothing into the duffel bag. Finally, he produced a collection of notes, written on small scraps of paper, listing items he had read or heard about or had witnessed personally, which were of special concern to him, and which he wanted to make me aware of. He allowed me to decide which ones to comment on, if I so chose, without any pressure to do so. Having in his own mind an expectation that we had only a standard allotment of time to spend together, he responded without perturbation, when I eventually indicated the end was approaching. Though he had more to show me, he graciously took his leave and departed.

Here was someone definitely attuned to aspects of the cultural and political world around him, who wanted to share them with me for our mutual benefit. Thus he established the format for how our work should proceed. This was not in the form of a demand but rather of an invitation; therefore, he appeared as pleased to be allowed to take the lead, as I was to grant it to him.

© Springer International Publishing Switzerland 2016
W. Tucker, *Narratives of Recovery from Serious Mental Illness*,
DOI 10.1007/978-3-319-33727-2_9

Over the course of our six years together Seth turned out to be a master of managing his symptoms in this way and of making sense of his life. He endowed our modest meeting space with the aura of a sanctuary and jealously guarded the moments we were allowed to spend there together: "That's my time," he would say. My role was just to tag along with him and to try not to interfere too much. It may not even have been much of a problem that I had almost no idea this was happening, right in front of my eyes and ears. There was no way I could have realized it at first, but we had embarked on a process that was going to help me formulate my own version of narrative medicine, long before I ever thought of writing a book about it.

He was a Caucasian man, 56 years old when we began, with short-cropped white hair, appearing physically fit, and frequently adorned with a comradely smile, though I was sometimes a bit slow in picking up what amused him. He dressed casually but always cleanly and neatly, usually wearing a T-shirt and baseball cap emblazoned with the logo of one of the New York sports teams. He described his interests as, "politics, swimming, rock-and-roll, [being a] Yankees fan, and writing." His manner was businesslike but also warm, as if to say, I know what is supposed to happen in our meetings, and you can count on me to hold up my end of the bargain; furthermore, I hope you will enjoy it as much as I expect to.

To put me at ease, he assured me, first, that he had not been hospitalized in 23 years; second, that he continued to be on excellent terms with his most recent long-term psychiatrist, whom he had worked with for the decade prior to coming to Pathways, and whom he invited me to contact for verification; and third, that he had been doing quite well for a long time on a low dose of a so-called "first-generation" antipsychotic medication, Stelazine, from which he actually had no side-effects, though he considered its effect in helping him fall asleep to be a beneficial one. He was grateful that this psychiatrist had relieved him of the "darkness," which he elaborated as being a "left-sided weakness" and "knobbiness," which he believed had colored his life ever since his adoption at birth. It seemed that financial issues were behind his having had to give up this psychiatrist, whom he was not yet ready to trade in for the kind of brief interactions that clinic attendance presumes: he still needed a more intensive therapeutic relationship.

Psychiatric and Personal History

Then he began filling me in on his life history. He was uncertain about the ethnicity of his biological progenitors, so to fill in the gaps, he appropriated many groups to his list, Scottish and Irish but principally Native American. He was raised by a Jewish couple, who gave him their name, and therefore added that group as well. Tactfully, as an aside, he inquired about my ethnic background. When I told him I was German-Jewish, he inquired further, "More German or more Jewish?" I replied that I thought of myself as more Jewish. "In that case," he retorted, "You'll have to watch out for the gas!" Could anyone who did not suffer from his condition ever say such a thing, so sympathetically? He had attended various colleges, but it remained unclear whether he had completed any degree program. He was an avid and strong swimmer and had served as lifeguard throughout his early 20s at beaches from Jones Beach, on the south shore of Long Island, to Hawaii. "I've saved hundreds of people," he told me proudly.

In his mid-to-late 20s, as I learned later from his sister, he suffered a series of nervous breakdowns and was hospitalized five times for loud, aggressive speech, in the context of feelings of being observed and of being sent special messages he could not quite decipher. Though shaken, he refused to be diverted by these episodes from his original goals: maintaining his independence, keeping up with the political and cultural life around him, and participating in events that promoted rights and services for those disabled like him. He dismissed the possibility of marriage and family on concrete, practical grounds: "Where would I find the money for that? I'm not that irresponsible!"

Let me settle immediately the question of his having a serious mental illness. Actually, Seth himself settled it, by telling me, "I may have a bit of bipolar, but the schizophrenia is the issue." You may object to my accepting his label at face value, since patients, along with the rest of the general public, use diagnostic terms like this to mean a wide range of disturbances. But Seth had had plenty of time to decide whether the label fit, and the evidence he presented in support of it was very consistent. His primary symptom was the notion of being under surveillance, as noted above. That cut both ways: he enjoyed some powers of influence, himself. For example, later, regarding the results of the U.S. Open in 2008, he commented, "Federer won the Open—I get credit for that," meaning that having grown up in Forest Hills gave him at least some bragging rights. Sometimes there was an intentional edge to this specialness, however. When he was annoyed at me for what he felt was too much coddling of a fellow-patient, who was also one of his house-mates, he warned me in terms I had come to understand clearly enough, "I don't play tennis, Dr. Tucker, and you'd better hope I don't take it up, because I'm from Forest Hills, after all!" As for the "bipolar" label, he knew what he was talking about with that one, too: he reported having quit an intensive day program, "because it was making me manic-y," meaning that it made him feel overstimulated.

Treatment

He would show up at our clinic for each monthly appointment, frequently ahead of the appointed hour, as our team's administrative assistant would inform me. He would sit patiently, not speaking to anyone unless asked, whereupon he would explain he "had an appointment with [his] psychiatrist." When I showed up, usually returning from a home visit to another client, he would routinely ask whether I was ready for him or first needed some time for myself, perhaps to eat my lunch. Only when invited would he enter my office and unpack his prepared materials. In the course of his reports of the past month's activities he would casually insert the comment that, variously, "Ambulances (or FedEx trucks, or taxis, or silver motorcycles) have been 'cruising me'"—that is, they had a special significance for him. I assumed that he was using that word in its literal, concrete sense—that is, driving slowly past him for the purpose of spying on him, perhaps but not necessarily with its sexual connotation. He would report this observation without suggesting any rise in his general level of alarm about what had long since become routine and now amounted only to a continual distraction. A few days following each meeting, I would receive in the mail an envelope containing a hand-written note hardly larger than a postage stamp and barely legible, announcing, "Good meeting. Covered the necessary topics. See you next month." I kept a whole envelope of these, and it did not take up much room at all.

Clearly, he did not need my help in accessing the range of recovery-oriented activities our agency usually suggested to our clients. These he sought out on his own. He wrote a monthly column for the client newsletter, attended such agency's social functions as its Thanksgiving dinner and its annual summer picnic, and traveled to the state capitol to demonstrate on behalf of increased support services for people with disabilities. With some justification he gently rebuked me more than once for missing these events myself, noting that I was losing opportunities to put in a symbolic appearance of support. He attended a College Fair at the Jacob Javits Center, an annual Earth Day in Central Park, a Mental Health Day film festival, and a Bronx MICA (mental illness/chemical-abuse) Committee meeting, among many other events. He had learned from experience that these events were more than mere distractions to pass the time. As he explained it, "I find that if I stay busy, I get clear-headed—I just have to push myself a little."

He was always engaged in at least one longer-term project, and no complication of it discouraged him for long. After he bought a small motorbike, partly in support of his self-image as a biker, he pursued getting a special operator's license for many months, only to fail the test several times, before realizing that an ordinary operator's license would suffice. In order to buy a small pickup truck to carry the motorbike around, he made monthly payments for nearly five years, before he was permitted to take possession, only to find that he had no real use for the truck after all. It took him nearly another year to find a buyer for it, and when he did, he sold it for less than the balance of the remaining payments, which he agreed to continue to make.

Most of the money necessary for these transactions came from his meager monthly allotment, supplemented by modest earnings from part-time office work in Chelsea. Unlike many fellow-clients he never requested a supplementary loan from our agency. In these, as in his lesser purchases, he appeared to be demonstrating, to himself as much as to us, that he was capable of budgeting his time and money himself, whatever the utility of each purchase might have been. Beyond mere capability he was also showing delight, like the proverbial kid-in-a-candy-store. When he varied his choice of which YMCA to visit for his swimming exercise, he justified the branching out by quoting a lionized figure of the day: "Coach [Tom] Landry taught us to vary our plays."

I gradually came to understand that there was a deeper meaning to all these activities beyond keeping his symptoms in check. I had noticed that he never spoke of swimming in the sea, which had been the site of his happy days as a lifeguard. Then one day, 4 ½ years into our work, he announced, as if to let me know more about how he organized his life, and how decisively he had put those days behind him: "The New York Supreme Court made it clear: no more beaches for you, Peaches!" He even made it clear that a typical month's excursions, which had included visits to Fountain House (Section "What Is Recovery, and How Does It Relate to Stability?"), the Bronx Zoo, and several more rock concerts, were intended to replace what he called the "real life" he had enjoyed before becoming ill. He summarized his adjustment to the new reality by saying, "I live a completely recycled life, thanks to Pathways." That these revelations, as much to himself as to me, emerged gradually, in response to many events, rather than all at once, would not be surprising to the old-time psychoanalysts among you, who have long been used to noticing the process by which guiding themes emerge only partially formed and over time.

As for Seth's paranoid symptoms themselves, he was in the habit of reporting them so casually that I generally restricted myself to letting them pass without further inquiry. Once, however, he indicated he wanted a more direct response, by announcing, "This surveillance has got to stop—the cops watch my every move!" This time, I pursued his question by asking whether the surveillance was so disturbing as to keep him from venturing out of his house to participate in his usual community activities. I should have known better. His response was to demur completely: "No! I'll flaunt it! It makes me feel wanted."

Progress with Socialization

Though he had no interest in intimacy, as noted above, and craved a space of his own to retreat into, he worked hard at socialization when circumstances required it. My agency's previous attempts to house several of our clients under one roof had all eventually ended in failure, with mutual distrust quickly leading to irresolvable tensions and desperate requests to be resettled in single-occupancy apartments. But this was not so with Seth, Gary (Chap. 2), and their third housemate. They grew to know and accept one another's habits and needs, and to look out for one another. When I asked if they would be willing to meet together regularly with me, in order to work out areas of tension or conflict, they readily consented. For more than a year we convened monthly for an hour in their living room. Gary would regularly answer my knock and let me in, the doorbell having long since malfunctioned. He then pulled four chairs up to a rectangular table, otherwise used mostly as a platform for figurines and various objects, since communal dining did not occur, while I went up the stairs and announced my arrival through Seth's closed door. The third housemate would usually be lying awake in bed but would respond, eventually, to my loud and persistent knock. Within few minutes we would all be seated around the table.

Usually it was Seth who would begin recounting the major events of the past month. It was enlightening to me to hear how his account would add nuances to Gary's, reflecting how his issues were with close socialization itself, rather than with control of impulsivity, which was Gary's issue. "Gary's brother brought us a turkey, and Gary cooked it for us." Or, "Gary took some of my food from the refrigerator again, but this time it was okay, because he asked me first." Or, "[Their third housemate] has been driving a pickup truck for the [Yemeni] grocer he works for." This was a surprise, too, because I had no idea that this housemate even had a driver's license, or that he still worked for that grocer, who, he had told me, had moved elsewhere to start up a new store. Or, "Gary did turn his radio down this morning, instead of waking us both up at 6:00 a.m., as he used to do."

Because direct confrontation would understandably have been uncomfortable at these meetings, little was actually worked through and resolved; nevertheless, many promises emerged, for example, to keep the door locked to any and all intruders—especially, to Gary's long-term acquaintance, who was persistently intoxicated, drug-bearing, knife-carrying, and threatening. After a few trials and failures they managed to restrict entry to staff from my agency. Nevertheless, the prospect of resolving differences permeated their thinking all month long, apparently to good effect and mutual relief. This cohesiveness was to shine in their responses to the new policy our agency was introducing, and which I will get back to, shortly.

All along, Seth had been speaking out forcefully at a wide range of venues, earning not only acceptance but also esteem, because the views he presented gave voice to those of many others less articulate than himself. Therefore, I was curious when he alluded once day to his having decided not to seek the post of peer-advocate, the modestly compensated position that entailed being spokesperson for his peers around agency policies, a post that Maria (Chap. 7) had so much enjoyed. It would have been hard for his peers not to endorse him, given his steadiness and willingness to assume responsibility. Nevertheless, I never questioned him, taking his decision as a suggestion of awareness that it would perhaps have been uncomfortable for him to have to identify with conflicting points of view.

During our six years of working together there was only one relationship that became troubled to the point of rupture. It was with his sister, who was the one family member he had maintained contact with. Like Seth she had been adopted, and though they were not close in childhood and early adulthood, they had become so, following the death of both their adoptive parents, when Seth was in his mid-40s. She invited him for holiday meals and never failed to send birthday cards. She participated in family therapy with him for half a year, until he broke it off, for reasons apparently more related to the over-exuberance of a young family therapist than anything having to do with his sister. The suddenness of the rupture was as striking as it was immutable. The successful step she had taken in her own life, namely, to run for public office, was, in his view, "Against the law, because I've had mental illness, and it drags the family name into public scrutiny." The vehemence of his reaction upset her, because it reminded her of similar reactions decades earlier which had led to his decompensations. Nothing of the sort ensued this time, but he had made up his mind, and during the last two years of our work together his references to their relationship described it as a thing of the past. I resisted the urge to encourage him to reconcile with her. In the end he had his reasons, and I was confident that she, for her part, was not going to abandon him.

Diabetes Management

His progress toward greater socialization was impacting his self-care, as well. He had been diagnosed with type II diabetes in his mid-40s. As he described it, "I got rid of the psychiatric impairment when I was 50, but I have a residue: diabetes." By the time we met, he was suffering from a common early symptom of peripheral nerve deterioration, numbness in his feet. He was aware of the regimen he was supposed to follow, but his adherence had been only intermittent.

With this condition the process of stabilization is only too easy to follow over time. For this purpose there is, fortunately, an available metric, namely, the level of a type of hemoglobin, called A1c, that indicates how well a patient has managed her/his diet and exercise so as to keep the level of blood sugar within a narrow range over the previous three months. Someone without the illness will have a value for this type of hemoglobin that is lower than 6. Good management in someone with the illness is indicated by a value only fractionally above this number, and poor management can result in values as high as 10–12 or more. Even values of 8–9 can gradually lead to severe consequences, such as the need for limb amputations and worse, organ failure, leading to blindness, heart attacks, and increasingly commonly, the need for renal dialysis. So common is this type of diabetes among patients with severe mental illness—partly as a side-effect of the medications which we prescribe, that this hemoglobin value itself is sometimes taken as a measure of how well they are managing their psychological well-being, which, in turn, is what makes it possible to manage their diabetes.

Seth regularly reported his A1c values to me, and I duly noted the fluctuations up and down without comment, leaving the management of his diabetes to him and to his series of primary care physicians, whom I never contacted. I do not endorse this complete division of tasks and am puzzled at my behavior then. Fortunately, Seth never let the matter drop. "It was 10 last time, but that's because I cheated on my diet," he told me at one of our earlier meetings. Towards the end of our meetings the values were regularly where they should have been, just above the 6.0 value.

Overall Progress

In regard to both his chronic conditions he was moving steadily toward recovery. So, what did he need from me in response to his monthly reports? Mostly, I think, he wanted to be recognized and appreciated for the efforts he was making to carve out a new life for himself, one that he recognized was not the one he had initially chosen. There were activities he could no longer pursue, but his personal values had not changed, and he wanted someone else to appreciate that. To make a success of this new life, he needed to maintain the routines that worked for him and to adapt to new demands. Indeed, these continued to intrude, threatening to disrupt the careful balance he had established. "I crave stability" is the way he put it. He did not need me to give advice or offer suggestions. The final test of his success was not long in coming.

One of the ways Seth gathered up his past experiences and folded them into our relationship was to tell me of his continuing relationships with his previous psychiatrists. There were only two of them over a period of 28 years, covering almost the entire period of his illness. The first one he mentioned to me was the more recent one, but when he died, Seth resumed communication with the earlier one, providing me with his contact information, as he had for the more recent one. He reported continuing regularly to present him with envelopes containing newspaper clippings and souvenirs like those he presented to me. It was important to him that I be aware of this activity, but he was concerned lest I take offense and imagine him to be dividing his loyalties. Thus he reassured me, "I'm not trying to stimulate anti-trust."

Early in my career I had indeed felt threatened by a patient's continuing contact with her previous psychiatrist, and with the backing of a preceptor I contacted that therapist and insist that he stop interfering. This time, however, thanks partly to having grown up a bit, myself, and partly to Seth's tactful approach, I felt no such threat. It seemed to me that he was doing his best to maintain continuity in his treatment by establishing trusting relationships with a series of us psychiatrists, as circumstances required, and it was enough for me to be considered part of that succession. Moreover, I believe his main attachment was to the agency itself. This ability to maintain continuity, through changes in psychiatrists and treating agencies, would serve him well in dealing with the policy that was on its way.

Seth got wind of a report that he and the others would have to vacate their house and also move on to a lower level of services. "I have a lease through the end of next year," he announced, "and they'd better not try. [The third housemate] and I fight sometimes, but splitting us up would be a travesty"—meaning, in one gulp, both a tragedy, and a travesty [of justice]. But once it began, the pressure never let up. Over the next two years, he brought up the subject eight more times at diminishing intervals, each time occasioned by one of my team members' urging him to reconsider.

Call it resistance or paternalism, if you will, but my response was simply to ignore the signs of this impending change, even when my agency began holding periodic "graduation parties." But Seth, a champion at facing up to such a challenge, plunged into the range of concerns that would matter in day-to-day life. He worried that some clients might not be able to make it, that there were too many unresolved issues already at hand, and that he needed the intensity of the frequent contacts our team provided. Touchingly, he worried that he would be unable to keep a watchful eye on [the third housemate]: "It would be very hard to 'rat' on him [if he were] in Manhattan!" I managed to get them a renewal of their lease, but this time, only for one year, not the usual two. He got the message. He began considering which neighborhood he would prefer to move to. He recalled his long absence from any hospital, his feeling of well-being on the medication, his having replaced TV-watching with reading, and his progress with his diabetes, including better management of his diet. It was clear that he had decided he was ready and willing to move on, if necessary.

Now all of Seth's experiences and accomplishments were coming together. He had been through changes in psychiatrists before, and he knew how to size new ones up. He was comfortable with me, but he could see, accurately, that I was only part of the team and of the agency itself, to which his basic attachment lay. If they wanted him to move on, he was ready to do so, in part out of gratitude for what they had given him over the years. He knew that he could make a new life for himself, by engaging in so many readily available community activities that he was not overly dependent on any one of them, and that he could make workable attachments to those he found receptive enough.

What I had tried to offer, and what he continued to accept from me over the years, was simply a feeling of continuity, a sense that I knew what he wanted to accomplish in the aspects of his public and his inner life that he considered important. I have a similar need to process my own experiences similarly, and though it was not within our compact that I use him in this way, I suspect that he knew this about me, and if so, he had certainly done his part.

Post-script

Since I did not know where Seth was receiving supported housing services or have direct contact information, it was fortunate that I had retained the telephone number of his sister from the time of our one meeting. As noted above, they had not been in touch since the time of her running for local elective office, of which he had disapproved. Nevertheless, as I had anticipated and certainly hoped, she mentioned when I called that he had contacted her not long before. She noted that he was living alone, as he preferred, in an apartment in The Bronx, and had no telephone. She gave me his street address, to which I promptly sent a note, requesting that he get in touch with me and explaining the reason for my request. He responded enthusiastically, and after another exchange of notes, he suggested we meet at the NY Public Library, between the famous lion statues. There we came in out of the rain. He suggested we "take care of business," so we found a clean, well-lit reading room, where he proceeded to do just that. He read carefully through every line, making comments as he went along. "Yes, that's true," he noted in response to the description of his energy and intellectual curiosity, at the beginning; later on, to his recollection of Coach [Tom] Landry's comment about "varying [one's] plays"; and finally, to his having avoided depending on any single community activity exclusively. He updated the number of years since his last hospitalization from 23 to 33 and corrected my calculation of the number of years it had taken to pay off the loan on his truck. Most important, he reported that he had re-established communication with his sister, as of late this past summer. In characteristic fashion he brought me up to date on his current situation by explaining, "I'm still going through a period of adjustment to the apartment and to the neighborhood. The World Series had something to do with that: I'm not a Mets fan." Finally, he summarized our meeting by telling me, "This has been a trip to the past—and a successful one." You will not be surprised that he duly followed it up with more than one of his miniature, concise, and yes, favorable notes.

Chapter 10
Donald M.

Personal and Psychiatric History

Donald M. was 53 when we met, but for him it was as if his life had only recently begun. There was almost nothing from his earlier life that he wanted to hold onto. He had suffered from schizophrenia since adolescence. He had used crack and methamphetamine in those years, as well, getting into trouble with the law and probably spending some time in prison, but he did not go into details. The way back from that life had taken a long time, along with considerable effort and persistence. He said it was a Double-Trouble (i.e., substance abuse and mental illness) program that "convinced [him] to stop [using drugs]," and he had never gone back to his addiction. It seemed fairly clear from some of his later comments that he had also spent some time in Creedmoor Psychiatric Center, but he did not go into details about how he had learned to manage his schizophrenia, either. It was as if, having reached middle age, he had suddenly decided to change direction, and had no interest in looking back.

Now, except for his age he was just an ordinary college sophomore, who happened to be a high-achiever. How he had gotten from the one life to the other remained sketchy to me for some time, so lacking in details that it seemed to have jumped out of the pages of a self-help manual that says the way to change is just to give up the old, bad habits and replace them with new, good ones. Rather than press him about his recovery from substance abuse, I settled for recalling something I had noted over the years, namely, that it is sometimes those whose primary problem is anything other than substance abuse—even another mental illness, who are able to give up addictions more easily than those whose addictions are primary. You could theorize that those who succeed more easily may have come to the abuse secondarily, using substances of abuse, especially stimulants, primarily to deal with the dysphoria of the mental illness or of the medications they were prescribed for it.

He had signed up with our agency seven years before I came. During that time, one of our photography teachers, Pamela Parlapiano, had encouraged him to get his

© Springer International Publishing Switzerland 2016

W. Tucker, *Narratives of Recovery from Serious Mental Illness*,

DOI 10.1007/978-3-319-33727-2_10

General Education Diploma and had, herself, walked him over to York College, our local branch of the City University of New York, to sign up for preparation classes. This hand up was all he had needed. A teacher there had recognized his academic potential and had encouraged him after earning his GED to apply to college, where he had matriculated two years before my arrival. He had been awarded a $1000 scholarship for books and supplies. He had maintained a part-time schedule, so he was somewhere in the middle of his sophomore year, progressing nicely.

In short, the most important change in his life had taken place before I ever met him.

Well, those may be the facts, but they hardly explain his transformation. They sound more like the next chapter out of that self-help manual. What enabled Donald to change, I believe, was his inherent awareness of what he needed and his ability to find it for himself in the resources that his college setting offered, as I will get to, shortly. My role turned out to be reframing the options these resources presented, so that he could choose among them in order to work around the obstacles that would inevitably arise, just as you would have predicted, when he began to confront the transition from school to work.

Initial Treatment

There was nothing else in his life but classes and homework. As he put it, more than once, "If I have nothing else to do, I lie in bed, watch TV, and sleep. I do a lot of sleeping." As much as I was concerned that he needed to socialize more and to develop other interests—at least, to engage in exercise, he managed to let me down gently, either by ignoring my occasional forays into other topics or by indicating, tactfully, that he was quite content with how things were going, so, no thanks. This was especially true around medication, where, duly responsive to his reports about a 20–30 lb weight gain, I suggested that he might consider switching to something other than olanzapine, a medication known for producing this side-effect. "I'll get back to you," was his first response; "I'd rather not change now," came shortly thereafter. He had told me from the beginning that he had figured out that failing to take his medication caused his thoughts to become "mixed," his "voices" to come back, and his sleep to suffer. He had no desire to risk the return of these disturbing symptoms.

He had walked into my life so quietly that it was a while before I learned to read the latent messages he regularly sent. Our first summer he chafed over having to wait too long for the fall semester to begin, but he was not depending on me to organize his schedule; rather, he kept that experience in mind and made sure to sign up for summer school, when the next year's spring semester ended. That he then managed to get an 'A' in both the courses he took, one of them in biology, will give you an idea both of his ability and of the seriousness of his commitment to keeping busy.

He was always moving ahead, not simply marking time. Interferences, such as having to move to a new apartment, because his landlady wanted his room for a relative of hers, did not distract him. When he mentioned casually that the new space that Pathways arranged for him turned out to lack the overhead lighting he had gotten used to, all the help he needed from me in order to adjust was to arrange to get him a small amount of extra funding for new lamps. His facility with online study aids certainly exceeded mine, though that would not have taken much. He was inducted early into an academic honor society, and the best was yet to come.

There was a particular kind of teaching that he appreciated, namely, the kind that was both clear and practical. He enjoyed a class on writing and research that would prove extremely helpful to him, when the demands of individual classes increased, "because the instructor explains things clearly," something he needed to improve on, himself. In a class on public-speaking, he learned "to maintain eye contact and to use hand gestures." These were precisely what he recognized that he needed—skills that form the core of a rehabilitation approach called "social skills training," championed by Robert Liberman. Here he was, cobbling together such an approach for himself out of resources already at hand. Never did he ask for special consideration because of his psychiatric condition.

Challenges

But, lest you think I was just sitting back and marveling at his academic progress, let me tell you what was going through my mind: I was trying to get ready for what surely was to come, when he went out to engage in his chosen profession, social work. The olanzapine was suppressing his hallucinations adequately, but it did nothing for his negative symptoms, such as reluctance to engage and to volunteer what he was thinking, even with me. People with predominantly negative symptoms of schizophrenia can sometimes be difficult to understand for a different reason than those, like Seth (Chap. 9), with positive symptoms, such as hallucinations and delusions or idiosyncratic speech. The problem is that, with people like Donald, so little gets communicated explicitly, that the listener is left with only subtle signs to follow. It took me a while to realize that this was his problem, attributing his reserved manner to possible depression in spite of his repeated demurrals. But from early on I was concerned that, sooner or later, that listener was going to be a professor or co-worker or client who was going to be very puzzled indeed. In spite of Donald's resilience and of his awareness of his strengths and weaknesses, I knew that at some point and in some form, his self-containment was going to present a problem. As long as things went well for him, I needed to back off. When the inevitable problem arose, we got to learn something more about how each other's minds worked.

The first moment of some uncertainty occurred after he told me he had petitioned the department of social work at York to be allowed to major in that discipline, and the department was taking what seemed to me a long time to respond. I wondered whether they were trying to picture how this student, however gifted at academic work, would function as a clinician himself. But, two months later, they did accept him, conditional only on his getting an honors grade in an advanced-level course that semester. He cleared that hurdle without breaking stride, managing an 'A-' in a course on "Sociology and Ethnicity: Racial Categories in the US and Worldwide." Because he provided so little detail, I never knew whether he had drawn on his own experience as an African-American man during this course; later, when he wrote a paper on homelessness, I did inquire whether he had used his own experience of that condition: he had not.

Two and a half years into our work, now at the beginning of his senior year, he expressed his first concern about his academic progress, telling me, "I have seven or eight papers this semester and hope I can get them done. Also, I have to interview a family and to sit in on a group." I was a bit puzzled over his concern about the first of these, since he had already written so many papers, but I assumed that it was the image of so many of them stacking up before him at once that troubled him. As for the requirements for his clinical work, we had some discussion. Sticking close to home, he decided to interview his sister's family, and he asked whether he might be permitted to observe one of our agency's group activity sessions. I was delighted to be learning more details about what was on his mind. As you must know, enough "concern"—his word, however understated, for how he was feeling—can make most of us desperate enough to reach out.

I responded at first with advice that seems to me now less than inspiring, suggesting he just slow down and take one paper at a time. Then I threw in something more tangible, offering to help him write any one of them that seemed especially difficult. This was something I had done in the past for one of my private patients, who had gone on to graduate and more. Donald never took me up on this offer, but he made the most of the uninspiring advice and addressed one paper at a time.

The biggest challenge, of course, was how he would perform in his internships, those practical experiences where he would be asked to function as a clinician. To my relief, he managed, somehow, to avoid getting his first choice, which was to work in a substance abuse clinic. There, I feared, he would have run into levels of aggression that would have been difficult for him to handle, even given his personal experience with this problem and its resolution through Double-Trouble.

Fortunately, we never had to find out. Instead, he chose to work with senior citizens, providing "phone calls and home visits in a community where I used to live." This sounded just right to me: elderly people would be less likely to challenge him directly and could more easily express appreciation. "I'm learning what it is to work," he told me, "and I like getting benefits for them and making sure their relatives visit." He even made an appointment to speak about that career path with a former client of our agency, who had become a licensed clinical social worker. I considered that act of reaching out to be a step beyond his customary isolation. But he was not yet out of danger.

Most of his last year of college sounded to me like a low-grade nightmare. Though he returned to serving senior citizens in his next internship, the level of oversight by his supervisor must have intensified. "I'm having problems with my internship," is the way he put it. "They say I'm not assertive or outgoing enough with clients, and that I pull back into myself—that I'm unduly shy and have social inhibitions. I'm working on being more outgoing." Sensing that he was sufficiently anxious as to be more forthcoming than I had ever found him in our four years together, I asked why he thought he was shy. "I'm afraid I'll be ridiculed—by anyone, not just by clients. I was ridiculed when I was younger. People have suggested that I try to 'break the ice' and get through. I can tell when I'm able do that." Then I asked what he thought might help him do it more consistently. "I was doing well with the [assertiveness module of the] Wellness Counseling program here at Pathways, but I stopped going because I was too busy—maybe it's worth resuming."

Things continued to go poorly. The next month, he reported an evaluation that contained his first merely average grades, ever. This time he continued to elaborate without my having to press him. "I have social phobia. I'm embarrassed to open up to people, because I think they'll laugh at me," he explained, again. His supervisor had instructed him to "come out more" and to be "more aggressive, more talkative." I recall thinking at the time that the supervisor must have had no idea of how difficult—confusing, even—this expectation was for Donald, but perhaps it was better that way. The supervisor appeared to be accepting him as an ordinary student having trouble learning a workable clinical style, rather than as someone with special needs. Either way, Donald was taking the admonition better than I was. He continued, "As for the [assertiveness counseling], it was helping, but I feel I've been through it, and I've exhausted the whole thing. I don't want help—I'll just try to be more outgoing. It'll get better with time." I could not have mustered such optimism myself, and, anyway, it was better that it came from him. Under duress, he was working out his own solution through just that self-awareness that I had missed seeing, earlier on.

Our Interactions

Now his assets of determination, single-mindedness, and resilience were being severely tested. He reported his supervisor's conclusion that he was "not progressing, still too shy, his voice, too soft," and thus, in her view the internship was not "working out." He countered to me that, "She's exaggerating, because I have improved. I don't need help from you or the team. I'll be okay." Even so, his confidence was shaken, and he appeared discouraged for the first time. "I don't think I'll get a job as a social worker. Could I work for Pathways? I'd be happy with a desk job in human resources. It's going to be a long winter."

For the moment I was at a loss, wanting neither to see him give up on his goal nor to put even more pressure on him. So far, my psychotherapeutic role had been limited to presenting back to him for his consideration, all at once, the options he had presented to me, over time. But now I needed to throw in something new. Fortunately, when I rifled through my black bag, I managed to come up with one. I had heard about a peer-run job development program, called Howie the Harp, after its founder, and suggested it as an option. Donald took me up on it. At the same time, never at a loss for long, like any other resilient student he had already moved on to the next challenge. This time it was a course in which he would be assigned to track a legislative bill, which the professor warned would be "hard," and to lead groups. There was the usual array of papers to be written.

This time around it seemed to me that our give-and-take even had some play in it. For example, he asked my opinion whether "the need for having a psychiatrist at a social service agency" might be a good topic for a paper. When I, of course, said it would, he asked me to provide him with a typical psychiatrist's job description, which I was only too delighted to do. I said we were physicians who specialized in the diagnosis and treatment of mental disorders, either with medications, when appropriate, or with psychotherapy, or with both. For his part, he conceded that "psychiatrists are needed to diagnose 'organic conditions.'" And so it went. The more difficult resolution of the issues around assertiveness could be left to the outside program, soon to play a major role in his continuing progress.

The relationships with his only close relatives, two sisters, one in Manhattan and the other in Ohio, became a bit less virtual and more real. They had contacted him periodically by phone and e-mail to inquire about his academic progress, but they did not show up, even for his induction into the honor society. Now one of them invited him to attend her wedding in Maine, and later, came to his apartment to invite him to a dance concert.

The countdown to his graduation was beginning. He was back to getting excellent grades. He brought in a draft of his CV for me to review. He attended a jobs fair, where he learned about various venues offering social work positions, though, as a back-up choice, he wondered about applying to Pathways as a peer-specialist like Ricardo Moore (Section "The Pathways Model" and Chap. 2)—not a bad back-up choice and better than a desk job.

There were a couple of distractions, one of which was his health. He brought up a minor issue over a toenail problem, which I was able to resolve for him by my usual approach of taking a look for myself, as I had done with Gary (Chap. 2), and then a much more significant one over a diagnosis of Hepatitis C, which he had probably contracted during the period in his life when he was living dangerously, though, in contrast to Bernardo's response to the same infection (Chap. 4), Donald's liver function had not been compromised. Fortunately, it did not require anything more, at least during the time we met.

The other distraction involved some of the usual administrative intrusions by our agency. Lack of help from Pathways' financial services for one month was somehow enough to bring about the inactivation of his Medicaid; again, he remained unruffled, noting that his past hospitalization at Creedmoor, a NYS-OMH psychiatric facility, made him eligible to reactivate his Medicaid, when he needed to. Urged on by our new policy of discharges, he agreed to a transfer to supported housing services, but he asked if we could continue meeting, "because I'm used to you." I agreed to continue meeting with him during the transition, which was to last another year.

The more important development during this last period of our meetings was his participation in Howie the Harp. I had suggested it to him earlier, when his confidence in finding appropriate work was flagging, and he had responded a month later, by asking me for a recommendation letter. He found the first visit there so encouraging that he told me, as if in gratitude for the suggestion, "It was good seeing you today." I was struck by his having taken me up on a suggestion I remembered making only once, in contrast to my usual experience—and probably, yours as well—of having to make a suggestion many times before a patient considers it seriously. Even when he learned that the requirement for participation was agreement to attend 95 % of meetings over the full six-month period, he was undeterred. As if in response to what I was thinking, he told me, "at Howie the Harp, they give us tips on assertiveness."

He bounced in one day to announce, triumphantly, "I've finally graduated, and I'm *summa cum laude*, too!" His optimism had been affirmed, once again. He had found himself a new psychiatrist to have on hand through his job search and thereafter. He was off on yet another internship, assuring me that he was already managing to lead a group. When I expressed concern that such groups "could be pretty lively," he shot back that he had already found his to be "pretty laid-back." It seemed we were back to our original relationship: I did the worrying for both of us, and he did the reassuring.

Post-script

I was completely without contact information for Donald. We had met only at the Pathways site or in the community and had had no occasion to speak by telephone. I thought about reaching him through his sister, in Maine, whose wedding he had attended, but I did not know her married name. I realized that his had been one of the few apartments I had never felt the need to visit. I figured my one lead was Howie the Harp, the employment service agency he had used to such good effect for six months during the last year of our work together. The administration there followed protocol, appropriately protecting his contact information but agreeing to send my letter of request for consent to him to the last address they had on record. Though they confirmed having sent it, I never received a response from him. Then I reconsidered and resorted to what many of you would have consulted first: an Internet search. To my delight, he was listed as a wellness-specialist for another of the agencies, Services for the Underserved, which had taken over some of the Pathways teams. I was able to reach him at his office, and he requested that I e-mail him my narrative, rather than our meeting face-to-face. As you may imagine, I eagerly awaited his response. I did not have to wait long, and when it came, it could not have been more gratifying. He had a few factual corrections for me, but he concurred with my overall picture, in particular, my emphasis that he had "negative" symptoms. He reported having been at his present position for the past year, and with the same agency for two. He said he needed to think over my request to return the consent form, but this, too, was forthcoming in timely fashion. His ease with the Internet certainly exceeded mine. But he had never doubted that things would work out for him, had he?

Chapter 11
Carl Z.

Introduction: Personal and Psychiatric History

When I first met Carl Z., a Caucasian man of 70, he was a semi-retired accountant, supported primarily by Social Security, and was a long-time member of an opera company, still very active as a singer. Though twice divorced, he was in touch with both ex-wives and even on good terms with the second one. He was in regular contact with his four adult children, three of whom lived nearby, and he very much enjoyed the time he spent with each of them. His life was full, and you would have thought he had good reason to take care of himself.

There was no doubt in his mind that he suffered from bipolar I disorder, mixed type. He was quite familiar with the symptoms and course of this illness, because his mother had been diagnosed with it, as had her father, who had ultimately committed suicide. This form of bipolar disorder includes episodes in which he would switch from mania to depression in the course of each episode, and each episode required a lengthy hospitalization. The first one occurred when he was 28, the second at some unspecified age thereafter, the third when he was 58, and the fourth, lasting five months, just prior to his joining our agency. On this last occasion, he required eleven electroshock treatments to bring him back from his severe depression.

As severe as his symptoms were, and as drastic as the treatments they called for had been, dealing with his mental illness was never his main preoccupation. Once again, when we first met, just after recovery from another severe episode, it had receded into the background. His focus remained elsewhere, much as Maria's did (Chap. 7), though for very different reasons. I was to remain in the dark about what these were, for quite a while.

Over the course of our meetings he came to speculate about the circumstances leading to his relapses, but the immediate cause, each time, was that he had discontinued his mood-stabilizing medication. All of his children worried about this pattern, and one daughter, a physician, astutely described his early warning signs.

© Springer International Publishing Switzerland 2016
W. Tucker, *Narratives of Recovery from Serious Mental Illness*,
DOI 10.1007/978-3-319-33727-2_11

But all their efforts, and his own, changing explanations, begged the obvious question: why run this risk, even intermittently, when there was so much to enjoy in his everyday life, and when the cost of relapse was so high?

Treatment

At our first meeting, he explained that, leading up to the recent hospitalization, he had felt "alone and depressed to the point of tears, unable to get along without marijuana and cocaine." When I then asked what we could do for him to prevent the recurrence of such a degree of misery, he replied, "You could provide me with an apartment; whatever else, I don't know." He explained that he had directed a production of an Italian opera the past summer, but he wavered as to whether it was his marijuana abuse or the excitement of the opera preparations that had led to his falling ill. He emended his initial request only slightly with "I'm a marijuana addict, so you could help me if I felt weak and tempted. I'm not sure I don't need someone like you to bounce things off of." That felt like a rejection of the offer to help him consider his risky behavior in more depth: things did not add up.

It turned out to be a good thing that, at his request, we were to meet three times a month for our first year, giving me a chance to get the feel of his life, and giving him the chance to size me up. On the one hand, he consistently presented himself in a polite, cooperative, and engaged manner, focusing with me on life issues that mattered to him. On the other, he invariably exuded a restless energy, and his invariably tousled white hair suggested he had just returned from a fight. He seemed always to have a focus of irritation or concern, even when things were going well, which they did, most of the time. For example, he began worrying about his youngest daughter's opportunity for an experience with the Peace Corps, over half a year before her departure date, and in fact, she never left.

Our first order of business was to change his mood-stabilizing medication. The olanzapine he had also been prescribed on his recent hospitalization made him feel overly sedated, especially during the morning, and brought on a 25-pound weight gain. We were in full agreement there, since both of us preferred at least a trial of lithium. He was so determined for it to succeed that he overrode my concerns about his initial nausea and vomiting, and later, mild hand tremor, attributing the former to a cold and insisting the latter had pre-dated taking the lithium. "Anyway, it never shows up when I'm performing," he insisted. As it turned out, he was correct about its advantages to him and to its drawbacks being minor.

Still, he made the change in his own personal style. After checking his cardiac and renal status with his primary care doctor, I had set up a cross-taper, planning to diminish the olanzapine gradually, but he abruptly stopped taking it on the day we had discussed the change. Still, his style worked out: he reached a therapeutic blood level of lithium without incident, and lost 13 of his extra pounds in two months. Thereafter, medication did not even arise as a topic of conversation: he was pleased with how he felt and took it faithfully, as the regular blood-level monitoring indicated. You are probably thinking that he must have shared my bias in favor of lithium for bipolar disorder, and, depending on your experience, you might not even consider it a bias.

After six months, his mood was already showing signs of stabilizing. He insisted he "[felt] good enjoying the simple life: watching TV and movies." He insisted he had no regrets about having given up his position as a tenured professor of accounting, although his private practice was dwindling. He noted that he was getting out into his neighborhood daily and feeling it was "more congenial: I've even found a nook of restaurants and stores." As he put it, "I don't have to prove myself any more. I've come to accept that whatever I can accomplish in life is behind me. I was a pretty good softball first-baseman and relief pitcher, and a pretty good CPA and accounting teacher at a couple of local colleges." He even began taking better care of himself: he underwent laser surgery for urinary blockage brought on by an enlarged prostate and recovered with hardly a mention of the event.

Still, when there were rumblings, I was not yet sure what to make of them or where they originated in his life story. When I checked his kidney function, as part of the monitoring of his response to lithium, and told him the values were normal, he noted that Bobby Fisher had died of renal failure. I only hoped his equanimity would carry him through, until the next set of rehearsals began.

Family

His contact with each of his children was so regular and so gratifying to him, that it would have taken considerable resistance on my part not to have involved them in his care. My first contact was with his physician-daughter, to ask that she check him for tremors or gait disturbances, each an early warning sign of lithium toxicity. Their collective hunch was that social isolation was one of the factors that precipitated his relapses, and there was clearly affection mixed in with their concern.

Prior to joining our agency he had lived with his youngest daughter because of his constrained financial circumstances. He admired her singing greatly, and she sang opera along with him, so he was relieved when she managed to postpone her plan to join the Peace Corps in favor of a full-time museum position in New York and a new boyfriend. Before this postponement he had responded to a news report of violence toward animals in one of the Central American countries she might have been assigned to, and he even reported a frightening dream, stimulated by reading that New Guinea, another possible posting, was home to dangerous rats.

He attended baseball games regularly with his son, with whom he celebrated Father's Day with great pleasure. He made a weekend trip to Florida to check up on his middle daughter, whom he otherwise contacted only by phone. He reported regularly at our meetings on his exchanges with the four of them, as well as with his two former wives and with an old friend. Thus, it was unlikely, either that he was unduly lonely, or that any signs of relapse to mania would have gone unnoticed.

These, according to the physician-daughter, included increased anxiety, a more disheveled appearance, and "being just a little off." Over time, their silence on the emergence of these signs was increasingly reassuring.

Early Life Issues

Now, we can get back to how he came to discontinue taking medication periodically, which, as it happened, helped explain the disconnection between his assurances of enjoying the quiet life and his simultaneously restless manner. Here, things get complicated: temperament, life experiences, and priorities all played a role. A year and a half into our meetings, he told me that he had been born Carlos Z., both clearly Latino names, in Cuba, son of a short-order cook. He had experienced the rough life of the streets while growing up, including having had a gun put to his head for having used the word "punks" to describe members of a gang he was trying to dissuade a friend from joining. He claimed that he had only anglicized his name in order to mollify his first wife's parents, who did not approve of his Latino background; however, I wondered to myself whether that change was also part of his transformation into a middle-class professional man of considerable culture, who managed along the way to provide stability and opportunity for his children. His youthful toughness had remained a source of pride.

Sometime later, in the course of our meetings, he made an emergency trip to Florida to attend the bedside of a younger sister, who had suffered a sudden heart attack. On this occasion, she recalled his having bravely protected her and a girl-friend, when they were all adolescents, from being assaulted by a gang. "I could help her then, but I couldn't do that now," was his commentary to me on her grateful recollection.

Opportunity for Change

Not surprisingly, vestiges of his restless and combative personality had remained. They threatened to disrupt his immersion in the principal organizing activity of his current life, namely, anticipating, rehearsing, performing, and sometimes directing opera. He speculated that the precipitant of his relapse the summer before we had met was the success of his directing performances of the Italian opera in a church, because it left him elated, not because it put him under pressure. His wistful speculation that all his life was behind him rang hollow, and it was not clear how well he accepted that his voice would not sustain major singing roles any more.

Indeed, he had not put his early life entirely behind him, and his equanimity was not unshakable: performance and recognition were still everything to him. One day he expressed severe disappointment at the opera company director's having passed him over for a small solo role. Immediately, he attributed this to bias, which he attributed to having attended outside acting classes, shortly after having joined the company. "This hurt me, because it's within my baritone register, and because I learn the score better than the others."

Not exactly out of the blue, here was an opportunity to draw on both my love of opera and my own experience with my demurrals and other's rebuffs of me (Section "My Personal Career Trajectory, Leading Up to Outreach Psychiatry"). I asked for more detail and learned that he had never spoken to the director but had only learned of not being selected by reading the cast listings. Not being any longer someone to let go of good things easily, I asked him why he had not considered confronting his director about what may have been only an oversight. "Because, if it was deliberate," he replied, "I may quit." The stakes were rising quickly, because, if he did that, his well-ordered current life could unravel quickly. Both his family and my team had noted deterioration in his appearance and slowing down in his behavior. Psychopharmacology offered no quick fixes here. I wondered what he would do, and I hope that, as you read this, you are on the edges of your chairs, just like me.

Resolution

Two weeks later, I had my answer. He had taken my suggestion and had asked his director why he had not been scheduled to sing the brief solo part, only to be surprised by the immediate reply, "How about singing it this weekend?" He was very pleased to be asked, but even more so, to be told, after the performance, "The solo you did last night was good." This was only the first of many such solo roles he was to be given, extending into the next season. His cheerfulness over this success then seemed to permeate all the activities of his life between performances, as well. These included outings with each of his children and time he volunteered each spring to help fellow-clients of Pathways to prepare their taxes. The negative changes in his behavior, so recently observed by his family and by my team, had disappeared as quickly as they had come on. It pays to have something more than a prescription pad in your doctor's bag, because even someone with a serious mood disorder can get depressed and agitated over disappointing life events.

That he had been able to accept my suggestion and to try it out suggests something more about his earlier relapses to mania and depression. It suggests that the final step, discontinuing his mood-stabilizing medication, had perhaps at the start of each episode been an active decision. Whether he made it on the basis of the irritability which is characteristic of mania or out of his characterological makeup, makes little difference here: he had found a way to cut the episode short without any change of medication. Would he head off future episodes just as successfully?

A nearly identical sequence of exchanges occurred around his transferring to a new psychiatrist. He was the first of my patients with whom I had broached the subject of our agency's policy of having clients move on to supported housing services at another agency, once they were doing as well as he was. He had responded in characteristic fashion, "In that case I'm sorry I'm doing so well." His physician-daughter's response was similarly pointed. She worried that a psychiatrist less familiar with him might miss early signs of decompensation or might not advocate for his early release from a hospital or, even more ominously, might threaten him with transfer to a nursing home, as his most recent one had done. Nevertheless, he asked me to find him one, and when I gave him her name, his only question was, "Is she 'into' opera?" When I followed up with her and could tell him she not only loved opera but also was familiar with the company where he sang, and that she planned to attend one of his performances, he was delighted. Their first meeting was a success. However, their second meeting almost became their last one: she had kept him waiting an hour, and he had walked out, not planning to return. Again I called her and was thus able to convey her apologies, so he decided to reschedule.

Regarding both these sequences, some of you may be growing quite skeptical. You may be wondering whether the psychiatrist here has abandoned his non-directive stance: does this still count as motivational interviewing? But I will counter that offering suggestions, or even intervening—sometimes, unsolicited—on a patient's behalf, is not the same as directing her/him to do something. Having had experiences similar to my patients' is something that unites us, rather than separating us. And in situations like Carl's, where it was necessary to persist in the face of criticism or outright rejection, not to mention, needing someone to intervene on my behalf to keep me from throwing away an opportunity, I had had plenty of experience during my tenure with NYS-OMH (Section "My Personal Career Trajectory, Leading Up to Outreach Psychiatry"). It may also have helped that, at this point, both Carl and I were at the same stage of our lives—the final one in Erikson's schema—yes, Erikson again! (Section "Why We Need Expanded Outreach Services")—and facing choices as to how we would spend it.

Carl had worked out an approach to his two careers, performing and accounting, that permitted some gradual diminution of commitment to each of them, appropriate to his stage of life. He had achieved a balance between disruptive urges and accepting support from each of his children, and he had no more than the usual concerns about access to his grandchildren. These were the activities and relationships that brought him comfort and pride. So, it is not surprising that issues around symptoms and medication never arose after the initial months of our meetings. He was aware that certain events or irritations could disrupt this careful balance, and he brought these forward before they created problems for him. He reassured both of us that, "I'd rather be here with you than moving on, but I'll be okay, as long as I take meds." The final gratification he told me about was that his opera-singing daughter might be postponing indefinitely her commitment to enter the Peace Corps. For the moment, at least, there seemed to be no provocation looming to upset him. But then there were his eldest daughter's concerns about what a new psychiatrist might come up with in responding to the next challenges that would inevitably come her father's way.

Post-script

Carl had done so well, had so much family support, and was so thoroughly engaged in his opera company, that it seemed reasonable for him move on to a less intensive level of support after a fairly brief period with Pathways. I expected to re-discover him actively engaged in his work and faithfully taking the medication that he knew kept him stable. Instead, when I reached his opera-singing daughter, who had pleased him so much by canceling plans to leave New York, I was sorry to hear that he was suffering from the onset of dementia. He remained living on his own, visited frequently by this daughter and by her older sister, the physician. I reached him twice by telephone, hoping to set up a visit, and he remembered me well enough. However, he explained both times that he was feeling acutely ill with a virus and asked that I call again later. So, on my third call it was a great relief to hear him sounding much improved. He reported having been diagnosed with lithium toxicity, which had cleared entirely. There were no longer any signs of confusion, and I wondered whether the toxicity, rather than dementia, had been to blame. This time he agreed to have me visit him at his apartment, and you may easily imagine how much I looked forward to it. When I called on the appointed day, however, he requested another postponement and offered, instead, to come to my office. You will not be surprised to learn that he did not show up. I continued with follow-up calls to try to meet with him but never managed to do so, so I have changed his name to protect his privacy.

Chapter 12
Seema S.

Overview

When we met, Seema S. was a married housewife of 50, living with her husband and two adult children; a third was an NYC policeman and had his own apartment. He had brought her to Pathways from the mental health clinic she had attended for two years with the thought that she would receive "more intensive services" from Pathways.

She had worked as a clothing store clerk from age 20 to 30 but had then given it up because of a physical disability: she was legally blind. Her bipolar illness was only intermittently her principal concern, but it was always her family's, because she sometimes became aggressive with her husband, when she refused medication. To her, family issues were paramount.

I could tell her story in three different ways, each one complementing the others. It seems to me that each version of it represents a layer of what was happening in her mind. Each one reshuffles the same actions and events. I will save the simplest version for last, even though it symbolizes and condenses the first two, because I was unaware of its importance before writing this story up. Altogether, it is the story of a woman who manages to put together an ordinarily successful life, by overcoming, successively, a series of very imposing obstacles.

Like so many patients with bipolar illness, such as Carl (Chap. 11)—Justin, whom you will meet later (Chap. 13) was an exception, she found it a perpetual struggle to accept medication, for the simple reason that she felt perfectly well most of the time. Consequently, over the course of our 24 meetings in two and half years, our exchanges over her treatment focused on her desire to discontinue taking it, or rather, to be given the option of taking it by mouth instead of by long-acting injection, which everyone in her family knew from painful experience meant she would skip it most of the time and would resume her aggressive behavior toward her husband. With me she raised a wide range of objections to the medication, from the possible, such as that it made her "restless" or that the nurses administering it at

© Springer International Publishing Switzerland 2016

W. Tucker, *Narratives of Recovery from Serious Mental Illness*,

DOI 10.1007/978-3-319-33727-2_12

her previous clinic "pushed so hard they drew blood from my arm," to the highly unlikely, such as that it caused her "hair loss" or "leg pain." It should be noted from the outset that she never ultimately refused a scheduled injection from me, even though her acceptance required many discussions between us about options and consequences, including several dosage modifications and my call, at Seema's request, to a previous therapist.

Besides this common issue around medication, there are two other generic lessons she taught me, though I should not have been surprised: one was that she was not only the one cared for by the others—especially by her older son—but also the one who cared for all the others; the second was that sometimes the dramatic improvement in the patient's overall condition may occur very early on in the course of treatment, leaving the remainder of the course mostly to reinforcement and consolidation. That was the case with Seema, though I was not aware of it until I looked back and began to write about her.

Version #1: Personal History and Family Issues

Though Seema S. grew up in a very poor country, Bangladesh, her grandfather was some sort of "businessman," by her report, so perhaps things had started off reasonably well. However, her father died when she was very young, and her mother sounded emotionally distant, given the absence of any mention of her during our meetings after the initial one, even though she, too, resided in the United States. Still, someone must have taken care of Seema, because she managed to complete high school at 16 and two years of college, studying "science," as she put it. At 18 she married a man 10 years her senior, and soon they had a son. It seemed as if things were looking up. Her husband, a dentist, emigrated to the US and began studying for qualifying exams here, succeeding with the initial ones. Two years later, he sent for her, and two years after that, he allowed her to return home to pick up their son, then three, and to bring him back here with her. That was the time she found the work as a clerk in a clothing store.

Then things took a turn for the worse. Her husband was unable to pass the last of his qualifying exams for dentistry, and he resorted to driving a taxi. She dates the onset of her psychiatric illness to this crushing disappointment. He worked steadily and managed to support her, their son, and eventually, another son and a daughter, who came along six and seven years, respectively, after their first. But money was always tight, and it became a frequent topic, first of their conversations, and later, of ours. When he once returned home to look in on his dying mother, he left her with only $300 for household expenses, and she asked me whether Pathways would lend her another $100, if she ran short, though, in the end he returned before she needed it. Another time, she related to me how she managed to feed the whole family of five on a budget of $500 per month, by running from supermarket to supermarket, chasing bargains. Touchingly, at the end of our work together, when she registered at a local mental health clinic, she needed to request a MetroCard, so that she could get herself there for future visits.

The financial pressure and the loss of status were grating to her husband, as well. He was frequently discontent, only settling down after increasing age and some health issues began to force him to, not long after Seema and I began meeting. Actually, the only time I met him was the day in the summer of 2010 he took off to watch a World Cup soccer match. He was in good spirits, perhaps because of the brief respite and the excitement of the match, and in that spirit he took a moment to tell me that she was "much better than before, when she was treated with oral medications, which she didn't take."

Even more a focus of our meetings than her acceptance of needed medication was her continual worry over her younger son. He found and lost at least a half dozen jobs during the time I knew her, mostly positions as a security guard, but he also prepared, at least, to become a taxi driver and, at the end, to become a clerk in a 7–11 franchise store. Between these, he managed to get himself hospitalized briefly several times for "suicidal thoughts." We spent most of our meetings talking about him or with him directly, notwithstanding my repeated suggestions that he take his concerns back to his own psychiatrist. She finally told me, "His symptoms are probably from me." Actually, though he may have inherited some tendency to irritability, the picture was complicated by an incident of abuse that he endured as a child at the hands of a stranger, which continued to preoccupy him.

This version, so far focused on family tensions, would be incomplete without a description of the very happy event that occurred during this time, namely, the marriage of her first-born. He had obviously gotten through the two years of abandonment he endured as an infant, and he was now an NYC police officer. He was engaged to a medical student, who would soon graduate as a physician. Seema claimed to have no worries about him at all and spoke highly of his fiancée, for whom she threw both a wedding and a big party, a month later. When I inquired whether it was to be a Bangladeshi wedding, she replied, "No: she's an American, so we're throwing an American party!"

She also managed to tell me her daughter-in-law was Jewish, a disclosure that in my experience—both personal and clinical—means the person has identified me as Jewish, as well. Here her recognition was soon to have an especially favorable twist, when, a bit later, the customs of her own religion came up, in the context of a discussion about her medication.

Version #2: Her Mental Illness

That gets me to the second version of her story, which focuses on what she acknowledged as her "mental illness." As just noted, she had dated its onset to her husband's disqualification from dental practice—a telling connection, even if also true. She was quite frank about her main symptom, describing it thus: "Sometimes I hear a voice telling me my father was Isaac Newton, and my grandfather was

President Kennedy." You should have no trouble assigning those grandiose family associations to a diagnosis of bipolar illness, just as her previous psychiatrist had. She genuinely feared the return of this voice and hated being hospitalized.

I had no doubt that she was sincere when she insisted that she was committed to taking medication, knowing that discontinuing it would lead to relapse, but she hedged her commitment by arguing just as passionately that past relapses occurred only when she discontinued it completely and assuring me she never intended to go that far again. Therefore, our discussions of the route of administration and the dosage remained a proxy for the need for it in the first place.

But even this back-and-forth remained very civilized between us, rather than deteriorating into the tension her husband's comments suggested. We even reached a compromise, in which I agreed to lower her dose by one-third, from 25 mg monthly to 12.5 mg every three weeks. She agreed that if her principal symptom re-emerged, namely, aggression toward her husband, she would accept the somewhat higher dose once again. She was quite precise and articulate in her understanding of the risks. She told me she was never free of the fear that the voice might return. "But if it does," she explained, "I'd think I was 'right' at the time and would be 'bad,' so you'd have to 'capture' me and raise the dose back to 25 mg."

We had worked out a ritual for my visits that was comfortable for us both. We never met anywhere but in her apartment, till the end, when I drove her twice to the local outpatient clinic. Before each scheduled visit, I would call along the way to be sure she was home and would not be inconvenienced by my imminent arrival. When I rang her bell she would usher me into her kitchen. She kept her modest apartment neat and clean, so I would offer to take off my shoes; sometimes she accepted my offer and sometimes not. All I ever saw were the kitchen and the living room beyond it, but there must have been several bedrooms, because, besides her younger son, I was surprised one time to be greeted by her daughter, a student at nearby York College, who was living there all along. We would sit down at the kitchen table and discuss her concerns about her younger son, often in his presence. Then I would administer her injection. Since her schedule called for these every three weeks, it was easy to set the day of the next appointment. Unsurprisingly, she never once showed the slightest hint of relapse: medication taken as reliably as hers is usually very effective for her condition.

Still, you would be wrong if you imagined that this ended the matter. Three months later, she once again brought up delaying the injection, this time, because she was fasting for Ramadan. I replied that Islam must surely have some provision for ill people—my culture certainly did—and offered to speak with her imam to get an official reading on the issue. "If you are that concerned," she responded, "then I'll take the injection, because all religions want what's good for people, not what's bad." Who would have wanted to argue with that?

We had definitely reached an accommodation. "Will you be at Pathways for a long time?" she inquired. I told her I was turning 70 within the next year and planned to retire then. "Will I need meds forever?" she continued. I was ready for this question. "Maybe not," I conceded, "when you turn 70, yourself." That closeness only made the parting more difficult for both of us, but you will have to wait for me to get to that, because first I have to tell you the third and most dramatic version of her story, and ours.

Version #3: Her Blindness

In Seema's country of origin, blindness among children was endemic. I recalled having read somewhere that it was ascribable to a vitamin A deficiency which caused the congenital cataracts to develop in childhood, but whatever the cause, she told me she had been declared legally blind from the age of 12. Some visual impairment must have been present even earlier. Treatment became available there on a reasonable scale only in recent years, as has been reported in the media. Having forgotten about these demographic factors, I supposed hers was an isolated case, and my lack of attention kept me unaware of the centrality of this issue to her life. What had she been doing about it? She had lived in the US for 30 years, had received intensive psychiatric care for the past two years, and, at the time we first met, thanks to her elder son, had even scheduled, but not kept, an appointment at Manhattan Eye & Ear Hospital for an evaluation. I offered to call the ophthalmologist on her behalf, but she did not take me up on it. Nothing had changed.

Then one day, five months after we began meeting, she announced that she had undergone bilateral cataract surgery during the previous week. This had resulted in good distance vision in her right eye; however, as she reported sadly, she noticed a deterioration of vision in her left one. But these changes marked only the immediate postoperative result. Over the next one and half years, she experienced steady improvement in all aspects of her vision, from improvement in her left eye, to (correctible) deficits only in near-vision, to excellent vision, near and far, in both eyes. At our last meeting she spotted the clear plastic needle cover I had inadvertently left on the table across the room. Her recovery from her profound disability seemed to me to have resulted in a great increase in her sense of accomplishment at having addressed a problem that had literally clouded her life since latency. The emotional impact of this recovery is only my best guess, for she never mentioned what it meant to her, but it is no exaggeration to say that what she had done by addressing her chronic blindness simply lit up her life.

What accounts for her having taken this problem in hand, not long after we began meeting, after so much time and so many earlier opportunities had passed? You can call it coincidence, if you prefer to be more skeptical, but it seems to me not uncommon that patients who find themselves in satisfactory therapeutic relationships make significant improvements in their lives, often without even mentioning them, so that we clinicians only find out about them indirectly, sometimes in retrospect, as I did. Did this dramatic change, which she brought about quite outside my awareness, arise as a result of her trust in me and continuing motivation to accept medication from me? I can offer you an alternative explanation, just to keep you from thinking I have let my therapeutic optimism carry me away: perhaps she took the crucial step out of satisfaction with the successful professional and personal career her elder son was enjoying. Still, it is not difficult to imagine what a very much reduced experience it would have been for her, if she had not been able to see for herself his wedding and the family party afterwards.

Resolution and Parting

We spent our last five months preparing and initiating her transition back to treatment at the Jamaica Hospital outpatient clinic. It was a delicate process, and I was not sure how it would affect her recovery, but in the context of our new agency policy, she had no chance of avoiding it. As noted, she had received only mental health services from Pathways, without housing, because her husband was able to pay their rent. As for relationships with other team members, she was aware they existed and sometimes welcomed them, but at other times she would not allow them to administer her injections. I do not accept full blame for this arrangement, because I did not aim for exclusivity and, in fact, I would have been spared some visits to her apartment, if she had accepted injections from other team members. Perhaps, again, her rather miraculous recovery of sight lay at the heart of my privileged relationship.

Unsurprisingly, her first response to being told about the transition was to request a return to oral medication. This time it was her younger son who expressed the skepticism: "I don't think she'll take it on her own," was his comment, echoing his father's earlier one. He redirected the conversation to the renewal of his musings over suicidal thoughts, but she was clearly upset about the topic I had raised. She bent down and began scrubbing to remove a coffee stain from the rug, showing distractibility that I had not seen before. Slow to catch on, I suggested to her son that this behavior reflected her worry about him, but he had his own explanation. "She's more worried about coffee stains. As an immigrant, she doesn't understand the needs of the second generation" was his explanation. Seema clarified the situation by standing up and drawing me back to the new matter at hand, asking me to call her previous psychiatrist, a Pakistani woman, whom she assured to me, would support her taking oral medication. I made the call but did not change course.

So things continued. She opened our next meeting with a request to postpone the transition, and not for the last time, either. "It's too cold to go to the clinic in the winter, "she said. "I want to continue with your visits until it's warm again." She reiterated this request at our next visit and again argued for taking control of the medication herself. "The injection makes my arm itch and swell," she complained for the first time. She refused the request of one of my team members to take her to the clinic to register, so I took her myself. She was pleased to be assigned back to the Pakistani psychiatrist, and I tried reassuring her by explaining that Pathways would continue to provide transportation to the clinic and would not abandon her, until she was satisfied with her treatment there. As it turned out, I could not back up my guarantee. My last visit came up all too soon, and when I told her it was to be our final one, she did not reply.

Post-script

Our relationship had broken off so abruptly that I was concerned that her commitment to staying well might have become frayed. If so, my hopes for the continuation of her recovery would have depended on her comfort in returning to the psychiatrist she had known previously. The clinic where I had helped her register was my source of contact information. The receptionist told me she had indeed continued to attend, though she was seeing a different psychiatrist, her familiar one having moved on elsewhere. Her new psychiatrist, a woman resident, welcomed my interest and assented to my request to ask Seema if she were willing to call me. She reported that Seema was keeping enough of her appointments and accepting enough of her injections to stay well, even though she missed them intermittently. She gave me Seema's phone number, and on my second try, I reached her younger son. He told me his mother had indeed continued to do well and said he would pass on my request that she call me. However, I never heard further from her; therefore, I have changed her name to protect her anonymity.

Chapter 13
Justin E.

Personal and Psychiatric History

Justin E. was 31, single, Caucasian, Roman Catholic, a college graduate, and a skilled graphic designer. Our interactions lasted only a bit over two years, but what he accomplished in that time was prodigious. He had fled to New York City from San Diego to be more independent of his family and to start his life over. However, he made four quite productive trips home during this time, and he never severed any of his family ties, which were in fact crucial to his stability. He managed to put together a whole, sustainable life for himself here, once he got past a very rocky and perilous beginning.

The story of his life prior to leaving his home town had many up and downs, not only in his moods. In his late teens, he worked for a year as an emergency medical technician and in the local emergency room. In college, he was a talented distance-runner, covering a mile in 4:45 and 3 mi in 15:30. I had run track in college, myself, and I can tell you his finishing times in his specialty were much more impressive than mine as a sprinter. His college career was interrupted at 20 by his first episode of illness, a severe bout of depression, characterized by anorexia, social withdrawal, and delusions. He attributed it to the death of an uncle who had been important in helping his mother to raise him, after his parents had divorced. It got him hospitalized and treated with electroshock, and it was followed shortly by a second, similar episode, requiring another course of the same treatment. After those two episodes he remained well for a decade, so that by 30 he had earned a B.A. in graphic design and had begun supporting himself by working at several printing and design jobs, though the longest lasted only six months. He also maintained a relationship with a woman 20 years his senior for nine of those years.

Arriving in New York without work or habitation turned out to be a disaster. His family came to fetch him, but he refused to go back. Then he had a third breakdown. As is not uncommon, his initial depression was accompanied, this time, by manic symptoms. Sometimes, such manic symptoms include poor impulse control

© Springer International Publishing Switzerland 2016
W. Tucker, *Narratives of Recovery from Serious Mental Illness*,
DOI 10.1007/978-3-319-33727-2_13

and promote frankly criminal behavior. He told me about several petty thefts, from a church's poor-box and from a restaurant table. The former was witnessed by a priest, and the latter, by the restaurant owner, who was counting it at the time. Both led to arrests and brief jail terms, followed by community service. Prior to these he had had at least one similar experience eight years earlier, when his stepfather had called the police on him. There were episodes of being caught for subway turnstile jumping.

He was e-mailing many women at a time, perhaps related to his mania. When I asked him whether he recalled having been manic on each of these occasions, he replied, "Sometimes I was, but not always." I would have given him more of the benefit of the doubt than he apparently gave himself. Fortunately, the judge he faced must have been thinking like me. He recognized Justin's behavior as driven by mental illness and sentenced him not to incarceration but to a forensic psychiatric hospital. From there, because of the minor nature of his infractions, he was transferred to a civil psychiatric hospital, where he remained for six months. On a regimen of Consta (=long-acting risperidone) injections his mood stabilized, and he moved on as quickly as he could to the hospital's transitional housing unit. From there he arrived at housing provided by Pathways. He considered the medication effective, but he was convinced that it was responsible for a weight gain of 40 lb, up to 290.

Family Relationships and Work

From our first meeting he lost no time in getting started. "When I have nothing to do, I get depressed," he announced. As was true with Victor (Chap. 5), Maria (Chap. 7), Donald (Chap. 10), and Carl (Chap. 11), work proved crucial to his stability. Justin's family knew of its importance to him. "We want you to work, even as a dishwasher," they told him. Within 3 weeks he had taken a test for a freelance position doing "courtroom graphics," bought an easel and a drawing table, and landed a job as a graphic designer and illustrator. He also considered writing a book about his experience with mania, so I suggested that he take a look at Kay Redfield Jamison's well-known one about her experiences with it. Though caught up in his enthusiasm, I thought he seemed simultaneously both a bit euphoric and on the verge of becoming depressed again.

Within another month he had settled down to business, working half-time for his biological father's pet-toy production company, designing and embossing characters on the toys and packaging. This relationship was to turn out to be the principal source of his employment. His father made demands that kept him focused, for which he paid him a base wage of $1200 a month, sometimes much more, up to $2500 a month, when there were special, last-minute projects that required him to work full-time. His father also called on him to make presentations to customers, and his praise for good showings on these occasions boosted his self-esteem. "We hit a home run with that big retailer yesterday!" he told Justin after one of these. He was to repeat this praise, using similar words, after the last of these presentations Justin told me about, two years later.

Two other family relationships were to play a continuing and important role as well. The first of these was with his older brother, who both visited him in New York and put him up during his trips home, spending considerable time with him. The second was with his mother, a retired schoolteacher, who suffered from very poor health but was always welcoming. He missed seeing them regularly and always returned refreshed from visits with them.

His father's support and encouragement were essential from the start, even though his parents' marriage had been annulled when he was five, on the grounds of what he called his father's "perfectionism." Justin felt compelled to work primarily for him, because the creditor on his student loan threatened to garnish his salary when he had worked for another design company. Still, it was hard for him to plan, because the arrangement with his father's company was constantly changing. He never knew when the assignments would dry up, not because of the quality or timeliness of his own output, but because of the uncertainty of the company's finances. At one point he was taken off his regular salary and put on a commission basis, forcing him to look for outside work, in case he were to be cut off altogether.

His father urged him to apply for total disability status in order to have his student loan dismissed and twice spoke with me about certifying him. I put him off, while conceding his point that Justin required considerable structure, saying I would discuss this with his son. Justin did not consider himself disabled, so we dropped the matter. The clincher regarding this issue was that the U.S. Department of Education had accepted an affordable repayment schedule of only $50/month. To the father's credit he never pushed this point too hard. The third area of disagreement, this one even greater, had to do with Justin's choice of girlfriend, but you will have to wait for me to come to that. To the father's continued credit he eventually made his peace with Justin's choice on that one, as well.

There is no question about his possessing considerable talent; you do not have to take the big retailer's word for it. Both when the work for his father's firm was sufficiently remunerative, and when it was not, he took on work on the side. One time this involved producing a set of graphic designs for a wealthy musician; another time it was putting together a portfolio of illustrations for children's books, just in case. He joined the Cartoonists' Society of New York, which held monthly dinners and organized holiday festivities. I customarily ask my patients to show me their creative work and attend their exhibitions, but all I can remember is one small blue-and-yellow logo for a pet toy, which was eye-catching and playful, and I am sorry I did not see more examples. His assets went beyond talent: he worked very hard, sometimes staying up most of the night to finish an item for a deadline. That habit leads to the next issue, his illness itself.

Treatment

Missing sleep can be hazardous for people with mania, heralding or even causing relapse. A good night's sleep is essential. He picked up on my concern about this issue and continually reassured me that he was generally sleeping well, staying up only when he had to, in connection with a project. We agreed that the Consta had been effective in keeping him well for two years. As he put it, "It keeps me from getting depressed." Still, he complained that the injection was painful, and that the side-effect of lethargy was a problem. In-patients are often treated with high doses of medication with the justification that they are necessary in order to hasten recovery from symptoms, but such doses are frequently incompatible with active life in the community (Section "Why We Need Expanded Outreach Services"). It had now been six months that we had been meeting, so I thought it was time to try reducing the dose, in accordance with his request; after all, we were meeting regularly, so we would both notice the re-emergence of any manic symptoms. They never occurred, and he remained on this lower dose up till almost the very end of our meetings. Only once, early on, did he report feeling "hyper," staying up late repeatedly, and wanting to take trips impulsively. In the past these symptoms had preceded a relapse, but that was in the context of his having discontinued his medication altogether, something he had no intention of repeating.

His weight problem was more difficult to resolve. "I hate my weight," is how he put it. He had managed to get his initial weight down to 250 lb, but there it hovered for the first two years of our meetings. He considered asking his primary care physician for a diet. Then, he got it down to 225 lb by "eating vegetables instead of candy," and by "starting to run again for the first time in five years." He was delighted.

The premise we both accepted was that staying focused and busy was the best way to avoid slipping back into another mixed episode of mania and depression. His personal life played a role as well. Loneliness there was as dangerous to his stability as idleness at work. To combat it he had joined Catholic Singles on-line and struck up a correspondence with a woman physician, but "the conversation changed when I told her I was bipolar." If he had asked me, I would have told him to keep that to himself until he got to know the woman better. But Justin did not need my help. His response to this rejection surprised me: instead of being discouraged, he bounced back quickly. Two weeks after the conversation he described, he struck up a conversation with another woman, while they were using the neighborhood laundromat. They spent the July Fourth weekend together, and over time, they settled on going out twice a week for dinner and a movie, along with spending weekends together regularly. She turned out to be a gem.

She became very important to his stability. Like him she was a college graduate. She worked as a manager at a housekeeping company and was its union representative. She had children and was somewhat older than he was, though not by as much as his previous girlfriend had been. They very much enjoyed spending time together, and he missed her terribly when he was away on visits home, or when she was away on union business. Once when his plane back from San Diego was several hours late, he found her still there at the airport, awaiting him. It would not be an exaggeration to say that she turned his life around by giving him both the structure and the pleasure that made it worth staying well. As he put it at the time, "I'll stay in New York at least another year. I feel good. I'm eating well. The fridge is full, and the place is clean."

Second Condition

Now for the "second condition" I mentioned above. Shortly after telling me about her, he announced that he had taken her to a casino, where he had "blown a thousand dollars." Since he had never reported the symptom of excessive spending that is common in mania, I took this to be an independent condition, rather than one that was secondary to his mania, and therefore not likely to respond to mood-stabilizing medication. Instead, I suggested he look into Gamblers' Anonymous. Without any reminders from me, that is what he did, reporting to me sometime later that he was looking for a sponsor, which is a sign of getting serious about engaging with self-help organizations that address addictive behaviors. Even so, like most people with an incipient gambling problem, he did not give it up all at once. As those of you who have encountered these issues know, it usually takes a protracted period, lots of back-and-forth, and even a financial calamity to get a person to make a serious try at giving up any addictive behavior (Chap. 4). Once he managed to stop himself from impulsively taking a middle-of-the-night trip to Atlantic City. With great pleasure he announced, "I might have blown the entire $1700 I had!" But it happened again, six months later, and this time, he reported, "I feel sick in my stomach for wasting that money, and guilty when I think about what I could have done with it."

When he told his mother and brother of this problem, they were not nearly as disturbed as he had anticipated. Their response was only to ask whether he was taking his medication faithfully. He feared, groundlessly, of course, that I might hospitalize him for it. The bottom line is that it never took over his life.

The loss of his eligibility for Medicaid might have disrupted his considerable progress. It happened because his income exceeded the (very low) upper limit. I chafed, as would many of you, at the rules that provided disincentives to people suffering chronic illnesses for continuing to work. It would make managing the need for timely response and event-driven backup so much easier if a little flexibility were built into the standing offer of help (Section "My Personal Career Trajectory, Leading Up to Outreach Psychiatry"). Victor (Chap. 5) faced a loss of Medicaid coverage for the same reason, as soon as he began to accumulate the savings necessary for his sex-change surgery. Without Pathways' willingness to continue providing services even when not reimbursed, many clients would have been discharged, since repeated, timely proof of eligibility was often difficult to produce: mailboxes were often broken, keys unavailable, forms daunting, and suspicions rife. Nor did Pathways have deep pockets to fund unreimbursed services, so making such willingness the governing policy must have necessitated shortfalls elsewhere.

Justin went onto and off of Medicaid coverage by turns, over the years. Consta injections are so expensive that without coverage they are unaffordable. We agreed he would switch to oral risperidone, which is much cheaper, and which Pathways provided *gratis* for several months. He managed this well, but such switches can be quite disruptive for less stable or motivated patients. He also considered two other options for getting insured: the low-cost, Medicaid "buy-in" program, and particip-ation in a group insurance plan through the Freelancer's Union. Though neither of these materialized, he managed to continue taking the medication he was convinced kept him well, until Medicare at last enrolled him on the basis of his chronic illness, enabling him to resume the Consta injections. This unanticipated trial of the oral form turned out to be a useful prelude for what was eventually to be his preferred route for the medication, first, because it was painless and second, because it was more flexible: he could take it with him on his trips home.

Resolution

Two years into our collaboration, he announced that "Things [were] going great." His father had just given him the second "home run" accolade, along with another "big job" designing more logos. He had parked his girlfriend nearby, so that he could join her as soon as we finished meeting. She had just remarked that she could tell he had lost weight. His confidence was up. "The past two years have been the best of my adult life," he told me. "I'm taking care of myself, using my talent at work, and have a steady girlfriend." It was December, and he took the occasion to note that his birthday coincided with Christmas, so that its arrival invariably cheered him. I knew I would be departing in a few months, so this seemed like the moment to bring up the possibility of his moving to an agency that offered sup-ported housing services alone. That would also mean finding himself a new psy-chiatrist on the outside. When he asked me if I would help him do that, I already had someone in mind. She was a woman I had spoken with recently about accepting Medicare patients into her private practice, who sounded both thoughtful and enthusiastic. He shot back questions about her age, ethnicity, and competence, and I gave him my best guesses.

Over the next month I got reports from team members that he had been inquiring about returning to Consta, because he had missed some doses of his oral risperidone and now had insurance coverage again. It did not occur to me that this new development reflected increasing anxiety on his part, so I merely reassured him that missing a dose or two would not cost him a relapse. That is not how I usually respond to reports of missed doses, particularly from manic patients, so I must have been pulling back, myself. Not for the first time, it was he who reassured me. "Okay," he said, "the injections sometimes make me tired, anyway."

When we met next, he reported that he had met the new psychiatrist for what he considered a "brief, general meeting" and found her "really nice: I feel confident it will work out." He had held nothing back from her, not even his arrests. He described her as having been "impressed" that he needed only risperidone and not a mood-stabilizer, as well. But he may have sensed some dubiousness on her part, because he quickly added, "She won't change my medication to something that will make me tired or gain weight, will she?" I promised to speak with her about his concerns about these changes, but I never got to report back to him: this turned out to have been our last meeting.

Post-script

I had kept the telephone number of the private psychiatrist I had referred Justin to, and her office provided me with his current telephone number. As he later told me, he was also receiving treatment from the Post-graduate Center for Mental Health team responsible for patients in The Bronx. He responded with his usual warmth and enthusiasm to my call, requesting I send him a copy of my narrative about him. Very soon thereafter, he called to say he would like to make a few changes to my narrative and suggested a date to get together. In his usual lively and engaged fashion he called again with more suggestions in the interim. When we met, he greeted me warmly again, then told me he had at first been concerned that my call meant that he was somehow in trouble, before I had had time to tell him my reason for the call. Then he went on to provide some details about his life over the intervening 5 years. Sadly, his mother had died in the past year from the severe, chronic illness she had struggled with since her own childhood.

He told me an interesting event from his childhood that had not come up in our work together. It was that he had suffered from severe obsessional symptoms as a child, similar to his father's, but that he had turned to prayer and had been freed of them completely from then onward, by his faith.

He was taking oral risperidone regularly and had even managed to lose some weight by more careful attention to his diet. To me he looked as if he had lost those 50 lb he had mentioned as a goal soon after we had first met. He was continuing to work for his father's company, as well as looking for outside work, though, as before, with only limited success at the latter. He had not returned once to Atlantic City's casinos, even though he had long since stopped attending GA meetings. Money remained tight, and he was still living from paycheck to paycheck. He had discontinued receiving financial supplements from Social Security Disability and was finding it difficult to deal with multiple increases in rent and other expenses. Through it all his relationship with his girlfriend had continued to flourish as a source of mutual pleasure and support. It sounded to me as if he had made the new life he wanted for himself.

We discussed the emendations he had requested, including a change in his name, to protect his family's privacy, and we had no trouble coming to agreement over the other minor changes he requested.

Chapter 14
Second Thoughts and Conclusions

Second Thoughts

As I explained (Section "What Is Recovery, and How Does It Relate to Stability?"), this book is primarily about positive outcomes, and I believe these occurred in all 12 of the narratives above, even though three of my patients died of systemic illnesses before they could enjoy the outcome of their efforts. However, it would be misleading to end this book without showing examples of the ways in which interventions could fail, or without highlighting the risks that outreach psychiatry entails for all its stake-holders.

Do not imagine that the in-patient psychiatrist has any more control over the outcome by prolonging the patient's stay. In those settings all that the psychiatrist can accomplish is the remission or suppression of symptoms; there is no way to know whether such control will persist after discharge. That is why it is so important to move to discharge at the earliest possible moment, when the patient has initiated a favorable trajectory. Retaining the patient in a vain attempt to eradicate all signs of illness precludes the patient's contribution to recovery. It also fosters a dependency that can promote early return to the institution, thus creating the self-fulfilling prophecy that any discharge is too early. Recovery includes adaptation to living in the community for an extended period, and it may be uneven, irregular, prone to slippage, at times halting, and at times spectacular. The sooner it begins, the better. That is why outreach-plus-engagement services are critical.

In retrospect the Pathways pioneers were able to demonstrate considerable success to their skeptics, given that they had access at the start to many patients capable of succeeding more or less on their own, once they were provided with stable housing and linked to mental health services in the community. Occasionally, such patients still turn up, but in the decades since these innovative programs have proven their effectiveness, and have therefore been provided to patients with more chronic and multi-faceted disabilities, successes tend to require more time and effort. They have come to require another crucial ingredient, namely, creativity,

© Springer International Publishing Switzerland 2016
W. Tucker, *Narratives of Recovery from Serious Mental Illness*,
DOI 10.1007/978-3-319-33727-2_14

again on the parts of both psychiatrist and patient. That is where the agency's protective function comes in, and where the agency's own creativity will be tested. It must find ways to help its physicians meet the ever-increasing demands for productivity and documentation that regulations understandably require, while protecting them from excessive administrative intrusions, so that they can focus their efforts to helping their patients figure out and solve their identified problems in living.

Four Types of Narratives Without Recovery

The other half or so of the patients whom I treated but did not consider to have recovered are not represented in these narratives for a variety of reasons. That outcome is instructive in itself, because at the outset of treatment it is not possible to predict which unstable people will decide, effectively, to take charge of their conditions and settle down, and thus begin their recovery. You may think that this allows too much room for failure, but if so, that is also the case with outcomes in the treatment of any chronic medical condition. In fact, the possibility of failure to stabilize and recover is precisely the point: the physician cannot prescribe a successful outcome, because it is the patient who must find the route to success. Both patient and physician are taking a chance from the outset, even though the stakes are obviously higher for the patient.

To paraphrase the opening of Tolstoy's *Anna Karenina,* the narratives of success harmonize; the narratives of failure are discordant. We can see a number of different ways in which my intervention did not make a difference, or patients failed to sustain their path toward recovery. I suggest five such ways, appreciating that my list is not exhaustive.

The first group were those on whom I had little impact because *they were already on the road to recovery.* They had stabilized before I met them. An example was a white woman of 60, who might have found her way with traditional clinic services alone. She was among the fortunate few who had managed to win so-called Section 8 support, which guarantees independent housing. She suffered from generalized anxiety and agoraphobia, but these were relieved sufficiently by her medications, which she took faithfully. She required only supportive care and was among the first to accept moving off of ACT services and receiving her psychotropic medications from her primary care physician. Another was a black man in his 30s with borderline intellectual functioning, who also was quite stable, capable of keeping his apartment neat and orderly and of maintaining his general health, who needed only to be connected to the appropriate and readily available community program services.

The second group included those who appeared to be heading toward recovery when my tenure with the agency ended, but *who needed more time.* An example was a Caribbean-American man in his late 20s who had dropped out of college because of a paranoid illness, and who withdrew into the family home almost entirely, but who maintained his motivation to return to college. His persevering and supportive but quite worried parents accompanied him and me to the campus where he had begun his studies previously, to meet the administrator who outlined the path for us.

A third group were patients *who were just stuck* in behavior that was preventing them from having a fuller life, unable to manage to get beyond the limited pleasures they had in their lives as they were. Some of these patients were very talented, so the loss to society from their counterproductive behavior is sad. One of them, a white man with bipolar disorder, had worked out such a life for himself. The only job he had ever held was as a violist for the Albuquerque Symphony Orchestra, 30 years earlier. In spite of support in times of emergency from a loyal and highly functioning sister, he managed to get himself hospitalized for provocative behavior every few months. He would push for release almost immediately, though in time his reputation preceded him, so that being granted his wish was increasingly delayed, and, worse, countered by threats to be sent to a state hospital; he was once sent there briefly but soon discharged back to Pathways. Between these episodes I would meet with him in Greenwich Village at small restaurants we both knew and discuss his progress over coffee. Pathways provided him with a used viola, which he had requested, and our agency's head nurse, a young woman who also played, offered to practice with him, but he promptly lost it. His willingness to forego success was most pronounced around picking up women: he could not help being so provocative as inevitably to drive them away, right from the start, even though with a little effort he might well have succeeded.

Another patient I would include here had sufficient resources to avoid the confrontation that difficult alternatives demand. He was white man in his 50s with considerable appeal and social skills, who had a history of substance abuse in the near past but never relapsed during of our contact. He was quite popular among our clients and maintained a social network. He was presented with many viable job offers through family and through other sources that he had cultivated. He even made a significant progress in his personal life, exchanging a highly critical female companion for a loving and supportive one. Then, in what should have been a favorable development, he was poised to inherit a considerable sum from a relative, only to have it jeopardize his support payments even before he received it. I recalled all these assets and intended to include him in these narratives but, when going over my notes closely, was forced to realize that he had not taken any of the steps on his own behalf that he had announced and looked forward to.

Still a third man in this category was a highly talented Russian painter—so much so, that a well-known SoHo gallery owner bought many of his paintings for his own home and put some on display. But, the patient himself disappeared for months at a time, resisting all our efforts to provide him with a stable apartment and whatever supports he might need to maintain himself there. The gallery owner and I met once and kept in touch by phone, but both of us ultimately lost contact with him.

One more in this category was white man in his 50s, devoted to alcohol above all else. He was a Jekyll-and-Hyde character who was quite reasonable except when drinking, when he became quite belligerent. He would get job offers but lose them by not showing up. He was threatened with eviction so many times that our agency could hardly protect him. When briefly sober again, he would declaim against the unfairness he had met with.

It would be heartless to fail to acknowledge that there was a fourth group who were so overwhelmed by a combination of severe mental illness, socioeconomic deprivation, and *traumatic life experiences* that, in spite of a desire to recover, they could not choose, at any given time, to begin to do so; they needed more time. It is important not to blame them, as if they had somehow failed, especially since, at some future date, conditions may be more favorable. One of my patients, a black man in his mid-30s when I met him, had already been a client of my agency for a dozen years before I came. He suffered from bipolar I disorder with paranoid features, from severe crack addiction in the past, and from limited intellectual capacity. Perhaps worse than all of these, he was convinced that his earlier crack addiction had literally broken his mother's heart, as he knew he had done, figuratively: she had died of a heart attack, after he had spent on crack all the funds she had saved up and designated for his education. For all of that, he was a man of kindness, politeness, warmth, and good humor. He earnestly desired to better himself, and sought, for a time, to enroll in a training program to become an X-ray technician. Other genuine assets included the support of a caring, if distant, father and of a highly competent and involved aunt, who regularly kept an eye on him and was not shy about reporting her findings.

But the cards were stacked against him. Once we had straightened out the only real medication issue that concerned him, namely, the weight gain that his mood-stabilizer was causing him, and he had begun, to his delight, shedding the extra pounds, he decided to give up smoking. That led to putting the lost pounds back on. He responded, either out of disappointment or out of skepticism about the new medication regime we had established, by skipping doses of his mood-stabilizing medication, and that, in turn, led to a return of erratic behavior and two hospitalizations, albeit brief ones. After that, things never did get back on track. He missed an open-house for gathering information on X-ray technology, his resumption of smoking was a continuous financial drain, and his confidence in his ability to manage his illness was shaken.

There are surely other scenarios than these four, from which recovery did not yet emerge. Acknowledging that a substantial number of those with severe mental illness did not recover should not come as a surprise or even as a disappointment. Outreach-plus-engagement psychiatry, as effective as it is, cannot be expected to suffice in all cases. If anything, the problems still facing the "other half" should stimulate continuing evaluation and new refinements.

Risks of Physical Harm to Outreach Clinicians

Those clients too dangerous for us to handle presented a serious problem. Fortunately, they were very rare, but no one considering working with those with serious mental illness should be naïve about the risks. These definitely exist, though estimates of their rates vary widely. In the surveys I am familiar with, the general public believes that 70 % of people with serious mental illness will at some point in their lives cause bodily harm to other people, whereas the actual rate is around 1½ %, as long as substance abuse is not part of the picture. The latter introduces a large caveat, which, in turn, contributes to some of the wide variation in reported rates of violence, but its relationship to any other mental illness is complex and hard to summarize briefly. As a point of comparison, the rate for those without any mental illness is 1 %. The press then sensationalizes these figures to assert that the mentally ill are 50 % more likely (i.e., 1½ % vs. 1 %) to be violent than their non-ill neighbors. Unfortunately, the combination of anger and alienation, which produce today's sensational episodes of violence, are probably much more wide-spread but also much more difficult to study than serious mental illness itself.

In my first example of a dangerous situation, I considered the potential risk significant but acted expressly to prevent an even greater one. The patient was a white man in his 40s, suffering from alcohol abuse and agoraphobia. We had tried enticing him outside his apartment with offers of small supplies of benzodiazepines and with intensive psychotherapy by a psychology intern, but we never succeeded in getting him farther than into our agency van. He lived in a fairly respectable building but kept his own apartment in a state of filth and chaos that reeked on hot summer days. When he was evicted, as was inevitable, and we found him another apartment, things got even worse. I learned from another client that he had invited drug dealers to stay with him, and that one of them had a gun. That was too much. Our agency wanted to send in the police, but I believed that might lead to a dangerous confrontation. When I had once by chance come upon a drug deal in another client's apartment, I turned around and left, unimpeded. So this time, I could only imagine that violating our own rule might have harmful consequences to those involved, immediately, and to our reputation for independence from the local authorities (Section "The Pathways Model"), later on.

Therefore, though apprehensive, I proposed to extricate the patient from his apartment by myself; my team reluctantly let me do so. I knocked on his door, announcing I was coming to take him out and relocate him, knowing others besides him were likely to be listening. A woman who was the dealer I had been told had the gun, answered the door and let me in. I found our client naked and told him to dress for departure, but he refused, whereupon the woman graciously helped me get him into shoes and pants and escort him out the door. When I slammed it behind me and told her Pathways would be shutting the apartment down, she volunteered that, in fact, an accomplice of hers had been hiding behind the shower curtain in the bathtub. Here again, our non-investigative policy had protected me: I would certainly not have wanted to surprise a potentially dangerous person trying to escape notice.

My second example concerned a white man in his late 30s, who seemed to be doing his best to get involved in treatment, presenting himself at various support groups where he felt comfortable. For a time, at his request, I would meet him at one of these, syringe in hand, to administer his long-acting antipsychotic medication in the bathroom. Sometimes, however, he refused, as was his prerogative, particularly since he had no prior history of violence. When he began an intimate relationship with one of our more isolated female clients, we could hardly interfere. Suddenly, however, he developed a paranoid delusion about her putting things into his scalp when he slept, and he struck her, causing significant soft-tissue injury, from which, fortunately, she recovered. While our team and agency were debating whether he presented further risk to her, he abruptly struck out at our receptionist/administrative assistant and injured her. She was a young woman of excellent character, tact, and sense of responsibility, who had been helpful to him repeatedly. She was traumatized, both physically and emotionally, and missed work for several months. We had no choice but to discharge him from our care, and I did not hear further about him from the agency that agreed to give him another try. Inadequately treated paranoid illness presents a risk to everyone, especially in the context of previous violence, which probably should have led to involuntary hospitalization on the spot.

The third example was the only one that resulted in violence to me—though the outcome for the patient was not the worst outcome among my patients. It concerned a Latino man in his early 30s with significant early deprivation and a history of having spent over half his life in institutions, as well as of type I diabetes mellitus, but without psychosis and not requiring any type of psychotropic medication. I tried for an extended period to approach his issues about commitment to a personal goal by focusing on the management of his diabetes, accompanying him to an endocrine clinic from which he had been dismissed for not showing up. I was able to convince the receptionist to reopen his case, and he was given an appointment; however, he missed this and several others, and he eventually asked me to let the matter drop. He had invited an aunt to share his apartment, and though he hit her repeatedly, she stayed on and refused to bring criminal charges against him.

One day I learned from my colleague, Lascelles Black (Chaps. 2, 5 and 7), that he had physically assaulted our psychiatric nurse-practitioner, twisting her arm behind her back and shoving her out his door. I was quite concerned that the physical abuse was suddenly escalating. I said I would make an immediate home visit, and Black said he would come along. The young man welcomed us into his apartment and asked us to sit down, explaining that his aunt had left. When I confronted him with his unacceptable behavior with our nurse practitioner, however, he became agitated and announced that he might leave our care and disappear altogether; furthermore, in response to my inquiry, he explained that he would find someone to take his cat. In the moment I realized that the setting of the current confrontation was lacking in security, and in retrospect, I wish I had taken the trouble to review his initial history before setting out on this visit, because it would have made me both more circumspect and also more sympathetic.

Facing him, I responded that he must be aware that when a patient talks about giving away his prized possession and dropping out of sight, the psychiatrist will have to consider those acts as a sign of suicidal intent, and hospitalization may be in order. In the next instant he rose up, strode quickly across the room toward me, and, as I rose, struck me in the jaw with his fist. Though shocked, I was uninjured, but the confrontation was not over. He dove into his kitchen and returned with a large carving knife, announcing, "How would you like to get an injection!" Black stood up next to me, in my defense, and asked the patient to calm down, but things might have turned out very badly, had not the aunt at that moment emerged from the closet where she had concealed herself and ordered her nephew to drop the knife and let the two of us leave. "But he'll call the police on me," was his response. "Just let them go!" she insisted, and he did.

We did indeed proceed to the local police station, where I filed charges. Then I was asked to accompany two officers for an immediate visit to his apartment. One waited with me in the entranceway downstairs, while the other went up to talk to my assailant. "Yes, I did hit him and pull a knife," the officer told me he had responded, "but he had it coming: he provoked me." Then, the two officers, my patient/assailant, and I returned together to the police station.

When I got home from work, one look in the mirror at my bruised jaw convinced me to go for medical clearance to a nearby emergency room. There the attending physician concluded that I had not sustained significant injury, but that, in view of my taking anticoagulants, it was only prudent to undergo a CAT scan to rule out intracranial hemorrhaging. I agreed; the result was negative.

It took six months for the case to come to trial. During that time a thoughtful Assistant District Attorney had suggested I consider what a reasonable and satisfactory outcome would be, and I had concluded that some type of action-response would be appropriate, such as a period of community service, so that my patient would understand that there would be consequences for his bad behavior. On the day of the trial, while I waited to appear as a witness, the ADA came to tell me that there would be no need for my testimony, because the defendant had acknowledged what he had done, and the judge had indeed imposed a penalty, which, rather than community service, was to be a period of mandatory attendance at an anger-management group. "Judges don't go for community service," he explained. The outcome and the explanation were good enough for me, but when the patient later called and asked me to take him back, I demurred, as you will be glad to know.

Risks to Policy-Makers in Supporting Expanded Outreach Capacity

Ultimately, the decision about whether to expand the capacity of outreach services falls to makers of public policy. Cost is a legitimate factor in their consideration. There is today a general consensus that institutional care, whether in prisons or in mental hospitals, is too expensive; so is "revolving door" care in the community. How much less expensive is the level of community support I have tried to illustrate here? Currently, several states besides New York (Vermont, Pennsylvania, and Utah, among others) and a Canadian province (Ontario) are trying it out and will doubtless contribute data and variations on the model. In the late 1980s there was a carefully designed study of this question that looked at programs in Monroe and Livingston Counties in upstate New York. It included fiscal analyses by investigators from the Wharton School of Business, and it found that community care, including housing, could provide stability and good quality of life at a cost 30–40 % lower than institutional care. That figure seems about right to me. If you factored in the savings from more expeditious use of preventive general medical care, the savings would, of course, rise still further.

This backlog of assumptions and traditions puts pressure on those of you who are policy-makers that is far from trivial. You would need to consider that there would inevitably be some fallout from those rare cases that go sour, leading to terrible publicity. That means you will need to prepare the public in advance for such outcomes. They occur now. People with serious mental illness may act strangely or be otherwise unsightly; they may seem threatening; they may be disruptive; more rarely, they may take their own lives, and certainly do so at a greater rate than those without such illnesses; most rarely, they may cause physical harm to others, even though, if you give it a moment's thought, you will realize that someone with paranoid fears is not plotting to hurt someone else, but rather, wants more than anything else to withdraw and to be left alone; hence the low incidence of aggression toward others. You will need to anticipate that the press tends to seize on these rare events and to look for a scapegoat to blame for having failed to provide adequate care and treatment. The recourse of return to the era of asylums is never far enough out of mind.

Besides policy-makers, clinicians, and patients there are other stake-holders whose opinions matter in deciding whether to increase the capacity of agencies who provide community outreach services. First among these must be the family and friends of the patients, who at the least want to know where they are and that they are safe and struggling to get back onto their feet. Those I encountered during my six years at Pathways preferred to know that their relative resided in her/his own apartment, and that a recognized agency was checking up on her/him and working toward specific goals which they could review. By contrast, many—though not all —whom I encountered during my tenure with NYS-OMH preferred to know only that she or he was in an institution for an indefinite period of time, safe and secure, without any anticipation of their release. Next are the occupants of the other apartments in the buildings our patients occupy. They deserve to feel confident that they will not be confronted with either danger or unsightliness, when they step into the hallways outside their doors. I am not talking here about the issues around the placements of group residences, which pose neighborhood-wide issues that I heard plenty about during my tenure with NYS-OMH, but of which I had very little first-hand experience and am therefore leaving aside. Then there are the patient-advocate organizations, who have played and will continue to play a critical role in moving the treatment system forward in a humane and progressive direction.

Then comes the question of value. How important is it to all of us that those with serious mental illnesses lead independent lives that include personal relationships, pursuit of personal goals and pleasures, and, not infrequently, meaningful work, at least part-time—rather than being put away and, frequently, forgotten—or, just as bad, wandering through the streets and emergency rooms? All of us are stake-holders in that question, because serious mental illness touches all of us, either immediately or at very close remove. Raising it highlights the importance of coming to a conviction as to whether recovery is possible at all.

The outreach model can be scaled up but needs carefully crafted new parameters. Though we were not surprised by our agency's successes, and we supported the idea of expanding it by creating more slots, discharging our clients in order to do so seemed a departure from the original contract, which assumed an open-ended commitment. That the pressure behind the new policy mounted in the context of the recession of 2007–9 with the shortfall of state revenue is likely to have played a role. Certainly there was no understanding among our patients, when they signed on with us, that they would be urged eventually to move on.

None of this is to say that it is necessarily harmful for all patients to step down to a lesser level of support services at the right moment. But to pick it, administrative parameters, such as length of stay at an outreach agency, is inadequate: had the five-year guideline been in effect when I joined Pathways, I would have had to discharge half my caseload when I arrived. There is just no substitute for a close recognition of the details of the past history, of character strengths, and of family support in selecting which patients are ready. If these are taken into account, it may be no more difficult ultimately to succeed than to fail.

For some, greater independence and less oversight can be salutary, marking further progress toward recovery. Furthermore, all clinicians deeply engaged in relationships with their patients are vulnerable to wanting to hold onto them for their own reasons. As far as our baser motives are concerned, you may easily enough imagine why we find patients whom we know well to be easier to manage than new ones, whose needs take getting to know. I believe this sometimes contributed to the practice of keeping hospitalized patients longer than they needed, when I worked for NYS-OMH.

So, if there were a will among you who are policy-makers to scale up such programs as ours, how should we collaborate so as to maximize its potential benefits and minimize its harm? One solution follows from what I learned over a decade ago from representatives of Donald Berwick's Institute for Healthcare Improvement, when trying to encourage my fellow psychiatrists at NYS-OMH to reduce the number of their patients receiving antipsychotic polypharmacy (Section "My Personal Career Trajectory, Leading Up to Outreach Psychiatry"). It is to have you, the policy-makers, announce the goal, within whatever parameters you decide it will require, and leave the means of achieving it up to us clinicians and program-administrators. Once it is clear that we are genuinely being invited to shape the implementation of the new policy, you will get the attention of the innovators among us, and enough of the others will go along to produce success. Thereafter, what it will take from you to keep the new policy rolling along will be reminders rather than threats.

Then there is the question of where the psychiatrists and other mental health professionals would come from, if there was ever an intention among community psychiatrists to scale up the capacity for outreach-plus-engagement work. There is still only one long-standing public psychiatry residency, the one at Columbia, though others have sprung up in recent years at New York University, Case Western Reserve, UC San Francisco, and elsewhere across the country. But, training in community psychiatry is not a necessary prerequisite. Any psychiatrist excited by issues in public mental health might also come to it, after establishing herself/himself in more traditional roles. There may, however, be some upper age limit. Though it has already been five years since I left the position that led me to this book, I did not think even at the time I left that I could have pursued outreach work much longer, because of the physical demands it imposes.

As for recruiting appropriate staff from other mental health disciplines, it would not be difficult to imagine how a seasoned work force—in particular, those already experienced in institutional work—could move out into the community, if they had the motivation and the access to a minimum of further training. Not incidentally, they could be employed by the same agencies that employ them now.

Resistance from My Colleagues

As I noted at the outset, old assumptions die hard. Frequently, no amount of data will convince someone to give up familiar practices. A decade ago, I was more flattered than chagrinned to be attacked in a letter to a very respected professional journal for my having expressed the view that it would be worth setting forth a list of standards for measuring the success of outpatient treatment. My critic voiced the opinion that only someone remunerated by the pharmaceutical industry would assert the possibility of recovery at all. That view remains the predominant one, among mental health professionals and the public alike (Section "What Is Recovery, and How Does It Relate to Stability?"), not to mention the press. Recently, on mentioning the subject of this book to widely knowledgeable personal friends, I was still met with incredulity: they responded "Do you mean recovery is possible?" It appears that this remains a new story.

Recently I asked a group of colleagues on the Public Psychiatry Committee of the NY State Psychiatric Association what they thought the major obstacles would be to just this plan. They were not slow in responding. There would be great resistance, they all said. First, in-patient psychiatrists and other staff would be concerned about their safety. From what I have just described, this was not an unreasonable concern. Second, they pointed out that successful ACT services require a commitment to forging strong relationships with patients, something that is not necessarily required of in-patient psychiatrists, whose principal task is symptom-reduction, in the service of promoting discharge to outpatient settings, where stabilization and recovery are supposed to occur. This, too, remains a realistic limitation, one that would require a more nuanced selection process and perhaps further training. Third, they noted that barriers to sufficient community housing continue to exist. Here, too, they make a good point. It would need to be addressed at the community level, whether urban or rural. Without available housing, there is no "housing first." Fourth, they reported their observation that, where transitional residences existed at all, the residents living there appeared to spend most of their time idle or, at times, even intoxicated, not participating in community programs to any meaningful degree; indeed, so isolated were these settings and restrictive were their guidelines that such residences did not qualify for federal community-reinvestment funding. Here, too, their point was well-taken, but I would have to admit to being shocked at how far this last model was from the program I had been fortunate enough to land in.

Like them I believe that there is probably an irreducible minimum of long-term beds that may be required for any defined population; however, I believe that we remain today far above that number. A lot of work clearly remains to be done.

Conclusions

Keep Recovery in Mind from the Outset

Within the working definition of recovery (Sections "What Is Recovery, and How Does It Relate to Stability?" and "My View of How These Patients Change") the first issue deserving of attention is getting the process started as soon after the emergence of symptoms as possible. At the point when each person signs on to receive outreach treatment, it is not possible to know whether recovery, thus defined, will happen. As it proceeds, patients may sometimes be aware that the treatment they are receiving is inappropriate and even know what they would prefer but still not know how to get it.

Goal-setting is a process rather than an event, and that it effectively continues throughout the entire period of treatment. My impression was that I could have articulated each of these 12 patients' goals early on in the course of our work, and that they would have endorsed them for themselves, though they might not have used precisely my words. It is not clear to me, even now, whether more careful attention to history-taking and goal-setting would have improved either predictability or options, though periodic explicit evaluation of progress might have reinforced our focus and helped avoid tragic outcomes such as Gary's and Bernardo's. It was clear to me that the process of establishing them took time and could not have been rushed: direct questioning from the outset might well have been taken as pressuring.

Still, if the psychiatrist does not have recovery in mind, s/he will not likely recognize it, when her/his patient starts moving toward it.

Family Support Plays an Even Larger Role Than Expected

Supportive family members played an indispensable role in most of these recoveries. This contribution should not be surprising, since it functions similarly in promoting recovery from serious systemic illnesses, but the family relationships for those with mental illness have historically been more strained, often due to patients' fears, often not ungrounded, that their families want them controlled by medication. I had encountered these attitudes frequently during my tenure with NYS-OMH. The National Alliance on Mental Illness, for example, has historically been made up of family members but not of those with mental illness themselves, whose advocates identify instead with their own consumer/survivor movement. But while I was at Pathways, my experience was consistently the opposite. In all cases my efforts to involve family were repaid many times, even in instances where I was unsuccessful, insofar as the patients appreciated the effort and were hopeful, themselves, that ties could be reestablished. I was never asked by my patients not to contact their families.

The bottom line is that my recovering patients almost uniformly recognized their need for family support, and almost none of these families had given up trying to provide it. Both difficult past experiences and Pathways' policy of providing essential support services that made independence possible may have created some necessary distance on both sides.

Peer-Specialists Open New Possibilities

Many of the theoretical questions around the value of this increasingly mentioned role are difficult to resolve, whereas the actual outcomes are clear and convincing. Would peers acting in staff roles tend to over-identify with their clients and thus be overwhelmed by a tragic outcome such as a suicide? They might or might not. How does one monetize the value of personal experience with an illness, so as to set guidelines for peers' salaries? Reasonable people will differ. Should further training in a traditional discipline be required as a prerequisite for employment? Probably, but Howie the Harp provides an alternative. Such questions as these three simply disappear, however, when your experience has been with someone as invaluable and competent as Ricardo Moore, who served as an ongoing example of recovery and stability. But his success also demonstrates how important it is to present skeptics, such as some of you must be, with such a role model. Jackie Robinson opened the door to blacks in major league baseball, and Joe Namath showed that the AFC could compete as an equal with the NFC, but less talented pioneers might have set those now-long-established causes back for years.

Pathways promoted two other roles for peers while still primarily recipients of ongoing services, as noted in these narratives. One is the more formal role of peer advocate, representing fellow-clients at special agency functions, such as a memorial service (Chap. 6), and serving as staff-extenders to resolve problems (Chap. 7); the other is the informal role of providing collaboration and support, especially in rooming situations (Chaps. 2 and 9). Together these roles show the evolution of a position that, if represented as well as these did, and supported by outreach agencies where there is room to experiment, may well become more familiar and wide-spread.

Systemic Illness Can Have a Decisive Impact on Recovery

It would be difficult to overestimate the impact of major systemic illness in shaping the course of recovery from serious mental illness. Sometimes it is devastating to the individual (Chaps. 2, 4 and 6). Nearly always it is ominous demographically—in particular, the fact that the nearly two-decade excess premature mortality suffered by those with serious mental illness is attributable primarily to their failure to get even standard treatment for the usual causes of mortality, namely, hypertension, diabetes, and cardiovascular disease, all of which can be mitigated to some degree by appropriate primary care, leading to life extension. Yet, in other instances the effect of confronting it can produce favorable outcomes for both conditions, while leading to enhanced self-esteem and confidence. A secondary benefit in such instances is that the patient's management of major systemic illness is an excellent measure of her/his management of his serious mental illness, and thus can serve as a useful metric of progress to both patient and psychiatrist (Chaps. 3, 9 and 12). In short the new catchword, integrated care, is indispensable.

Engaging the systemic illness actively can be at least as gratifying for us psychiatrists as for our patients. It goes beyond asserting the primary identification some of us feel as physicians: it presents a practical, hands-on experience that teaches us something about the process and management of chronic or at least prolonged systemic conditions. I learned a considerable amount about the presentation, evolution, and resolution of symptoms of hyperthyroidism (Chap. 3), notwithstanding my initial embarrassment at having to be told by a young resident that I had failed to recognize this diagnosis. I was pleased that my confidence in Richard's reliability was vindicated by the fact that only a crushing illness could prevent him from keeping his monthly appointment; that I was able to figure out that his suddenly devastating neurological symptoms had to come from somewhere in his brain other than his cerebral cortex; and that I was able to use my knowledge of the course of metastatic lung cancer, recalled from histories presented to me by former patients regarding their family members, in order to support his desire for relative independence, up to the time of his death (Chap. 6).

Even beyond these specific gratifications, I found it exhilarating to find, again and again, when I reached out to non-psychiatric medical colleagues, both physicians and surgeons, at private offices, clinics, and hospitals in Queens and elsewhere, that so many of them responded in a welcoming and collegial fashion. Together we constituted virtual treatment teams, each of us invested in learning more about our mutual patient's overall condition and progress. Nor were these virtual teams exclusively transitory: especially in my home borough of Queens, I became a regular and even familiar figure in their emergency rooms and general medical units. What I offered was baseline information, housing capacity, and follow-up treatment; what I gained was contact with my patients and often considerable leverage toward their earlier release. There is no need to overstate my case: not all my efforts to reach out or reach in were welcomed, but most of them were, and finding like-minded colleagues reinforced my conviction about the motivations of public-health minded physicians and thus, about the unexceptional nature of my own.

Outreach Work Expands the Psychiatrist's Role

If it is true that most people with serious mental illness will eventually recover spontaneously, as Bleuler surmised in 1911 and Harding demonstrated conclusively in the 1980s (Section "What Is Recovery, and How Does It Relate to Stability?"), then what is the role of the psychiatrist, or for that matter, of mental health treatment at all? The short answer, I think, is that the purpose of treatment throughout its course is to help support the joint processes of stabilization and recovery, as soon as possible after the condition emerges, or at whatever point the treatment begins, to prevent enormous suffering and stagnation. The substance abuse treatment field, where it is a rule of thumb that heavy users and abusers either give the substances up by middle age or are likely not to survive, has long endorsed this role. How the psychiatrist configures this role depends on many factors, among them, her/his willingness to provide a service rather than being directive, and, importantly, the intellectual and emotional resources, along with life experiences, that s/he brings to the treatment relationship.

Accepting a collaborative role as a member of a team rather than taking on a supervisory one may be difficult for many psychiatrists. We are used to being in charge. We have had the most extensive training, particularly with the biological aspects of the bio-psycho-social paradigm, as Donald (Chap. 10) was quick to point out. But in outreach settings, our authority within a team derives not from our advanced degrees but from our demonstration of competence.

On the other hand, because we are the most expensive, there has long been great fiscal pressure on healthcare organizations to utilize us exclusively to formulate diagnoses and prescribe medications. This limited role has proven a trap, not only for us and our patients, but for the healthcare organizations we work for, as well, because we have also been trained to provide psychotherapy, which is the foundation of individualized care, and can promote effective treatment in less restrictive settings, thus lowering overall system costs. Fortunately, our role may soon expand significantly, thanks to the recent study by Kane and colleagues (Section "Why We Need Expanded Outreach Services"), which concludes with what some of you have long known intuitively, namely, that the inclusion of psychotherapy significantly enhances outcomes beyond what medication alone can produce. It is likely that this conclusion will gradually be implemented by changes in our role. Outreach settings, where flexibility is the rule, already endorse this option.

Meanwhile, once we psychiatrists can accept that psychopharmacology may be a necessary but not sufficient intervention for promoting recovery, it will follow that collaboration with other team members leverages our effectiveness by providing a range of services we neither could nor would wish to provide alone. My role only started with the traditional functions of diagnostician and prescriber. Then things got even more interesting. Both the working diagnosis and the medication had to be agreeable to the patient. That may sound reasonable enough—even traditional. So, you may be wondering, how is it different in outreach work from what it is in hospital, clinic, and office settings? First, we get an opportunity that you only dream about when working in those more familiar settings, namely, of seeing patients in their real-world interactions with other people. You can easily imagine how the spontaneous affirmations from casual acquaintances confirmed my impressions of Richard's character (Chap. 6), while I was wheeling him through his neighborhood supermarket. Similarly, you will appreciate how Maria's showing up in her shimmering, blue-sequined dress on her way to a gala sponsored by Avon illustrated more than any verbal expression how animated she felt by her new-found pride (Chap. 7).

Furthermore, I got continual feedback from team members familiar with aspects of my patients' daily lives that I did not see first-hand. I was, of course, familiar with such feedback from in-patient team members in my previous career, but here it provided glimpses into my patients' progress or crises in their daily lives, rather than only accounts of symptomatic improvement.

Outreach Psychiatry Needs You

Obviously, outreach psychiatry is not for the faint of heart. It requires a personal cost/benefit analysis from each of you. There are many risks, not only those relating to safety. You will need to grow comfortable with reporting to a team leader with less formal education than you have had. You will need to accept that you have to demonstrate your value through competence, rather than expect it as a prerogative of your medical degree. Your judgments will be challenged, and you will have to re-examine your assumptions, some of which will change. But if, as a psychiatrist or other mental health professional, you want to see how serious mental illness plays out over time in the larger world, and to settle these questions about recovery for yourself, here is your chance.

A controlled setting where people with these conditions have been sent is a good place to see a range of disturbing symptoms and even to watch some of them diminish or disappear, but it is not a good place to see what the people who have them will do next, if they are given a chance. That requires their return to the community, where they will either pick up the threads of their lives or they will not.

To do so, they require precisely what people without these conditions require to accomplish their goals, namely, that someone takes an interest in them personally and hang around long enough with encouragement and a few resources for them to access when they need them.

Now here comes a more personal benefit. Because outreach work is both physically and emotionally exhausting, you will need to be clear about your own motivations for pursuing it. Doing something useful and cost-effective for society will not sustain you over the long term. What will is having your own questions that you seek answers to. For me these were questions about the nature of change and about how it could proceed as the patient saw fit, once the acute crisis was past. You may choose to prioritize other issues, such as the different arcs of various diagnostic categories, or family dynamics, or how particular psychiatric and general medical conditions interrelate. The point is, you need to have skin in the game, or it will not be very exciting or rewarding.

If you want to play a role in this process; if providing individualized treatment is your goal, because you are convinced that each person's recovery is unique; if you enjoy practicing mainstream medicine and incorporating the relevant neuroscience and its applications as they come along, but always regard them with some skepticism until you have figured out how to apply them to the person in front of you; and if you happen to be curious about enormous suffering and stagnation and the process of change without having to believe you can control it, then outreach work is for you. Believe me, there are plenty of places where you will be welcome to start.

Index

CPSIA information can be obtained at www.ICGtesting.com
Printed in the USA
BVOW06*1832220516

449085BV00006B/15/P